EDIBLE CRAFTS KIDS' COOKBOOK
AGES 4–8

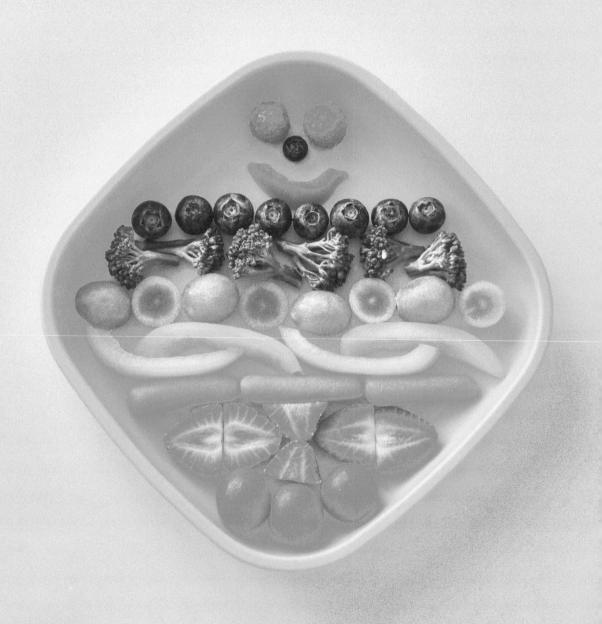

Charity Mathews

EDIBLE CRAFTS
KIDS' COOKBOOK

Ages 4–8

≥25≤
**Fun Projects to
Make and Eat!**

ROCKRIDGE
PRESS

For general information on our other products and services or to obtain technical support, please contact our Customer Care Department within the United States at (866) 744-2665, or outside the United States at (510) 253-0500.

Rockridge Press publishes its books in a variety of electronic and print formats. Some content that appears in print may not be available in electronic books, and vice versa.

TRADEMARKS: Rockridge Press and the Rockridge Press logo are trademarks or registered trademarks of Callisto Media Inc. and/or its affiliates, in the United States and other countries, and may not be used without written permission. All other trademarks are the property of their respective owners. Rockridge Press is not associated with any product or vendor mentioned in this book.

Interior and Cover Designer: Rachel Haeseker
Art Producer: Sara Feinstein
Editor: Andrea Leptinsky
Production Editor: Ruth Sakata Corley
Production Manager: Michael Kay

Photography © 2021 Laura Flippen, cover, p. ii, vi, xii-1, 5-7, 12, 15-16, 19-20, 23-24, 28, 32, 36, 40, 44, 48, 51-52, 56, 60, 64, 68, 72, 76, 80, 84, 88, 92, 96, 99, 100, 103-104, 107; © Darren Muir, p. 8, 11. Food styling by Laura Flippen, cover, p. ii, vi, xii-1, 5-7, 12, 15-16, 19-20, 23-24, 28, 32, 36, 40, 44, 48, 51-52, 56, 60, 64, 68, 72, 76, 80, 84, 88, 92, 96, 99, 100, 103-104, 107. Food styling by Yolanda Muir, p. 8, 11.

ISBN: Print 978-1-63807-034-4
eBook 978-1-63807-818-0
R0

To Violet and George,
my littlest foodies

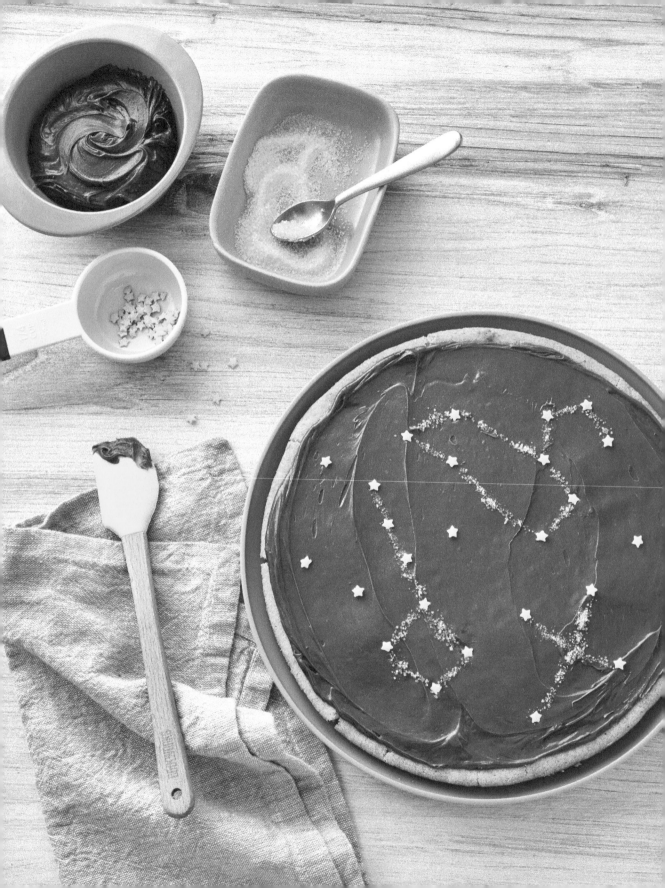

CONTENTS

A NOTE TO GROWN-UPS

If your kids are like mine, it's always easy to find them in the kitchen. My four kids often perch on a stool doing homework while I prep dinner, but on our favorite days, their little hands are busy with something other than pencils and tablets . . . they're making yummy food art!

Cooking with kids is a way to create lasting memories, but kids who are comfortable in the kitchen also get a ton of benefits in the meantime: a sense of curiosity, creativity, growing independence, and even a willingness to try new foods.

Approach each recipe in this book like a craft project, one the kids can eat in the end. (No need to supply a snack. It's built in!) You'll need to set out the supplies, but depending on their ages and skills, kids will be able to complete a lot of the steps themselves. Here are some additional tips to get the most out of these projects:

▶ **Set aside about an hour for each project.** Some recipes will need longer than that to either bake, harden, or freeze, but giving yourself a generous amount of time will always make the process smoother than rushing or wishing you didn't need to head out the door halfway through.

▶ **Fingers are allowed!** If you don't mind a little mess, this is an opportunity for kids to taste as they go. Most of the ingredients will be tempting, but of course watch out for raw eggs (of which there are very few here). Encouraging kids to develop their sense of smell can be fun too. I like to ask them about the textures—Does this feel bumpy or smooth?—and talk about our favorite colors and combinations of ingredients.

▶ **Let kids experiment.** It's only a matter of minutes before what started as a bunny turns into a turtle for one kid and a monster for someone else. Putting a personal spin on each project is part of the fun.

▶ **Since each child's skills will vary, you can decide which tasks yours can do all by themselves.** There's nothing like a tiny cook who can say "I made it myself!" These creations won't be perfect, so encourage them to run with their imaginations rather than worry about missing the mark.

In this book you'll find 25 snack recipes that encourage play and creativity to help kids grow comfortable in the kitchen as they gain cooking skills. Each one is labeled with a "messy meter," 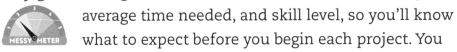 average time needed, and skill level, so you'll know what to expect before you begin each project. You know best what your little cooks are capable of, so set limits on what is safe and doable for your child. And along the way, you'll also find fun facts, tips, and suggestions for how kids can make their own unique works of edible art.

Got readers? You can turn them loose with a pad of sticky notes so that they can flag the projects they want to do first. You'll want to read through the whole recipe and supply list before beginning anyway. That way you can pick a date and time, rather than "right now," to make sure you'll have all the ingredients on hand.

I hope you have as much fun making—and eating—all these crafts as we did.

A NOTE TO KIDS

What's better than a cool art project? One you can eat too! This book is bursting with food ideas for you to make on your own or with friends or grown-ups. Every recipe is one that my four kids tried (and loved) so that we could write out the instructions as clearly as possible for you.

You'll find difficulty ratings—easy, medium, and hard—for each one, plus you can see which are dairy-free, gluten-free, nut-free, or vegetarian. When you see ask an adult, that's your cue to find a grown-up to help. Those steps usually involve knives or using the stove and oven. But don't worry, most of the fun is all yours. Look for the words "Extra Crafty" to give you even more ideas about how to spin each project into a new idea just for you. You'll see fun facts, top tips, and even some jokes to make your kitchen the most fun place on the block.

To start, take a pile of sticky notes (or a few strips of regular paper bookmarks) and mark up a handful of pages you want to try first. Then tell your grown-ups so that they can collect any ingredients or supplies they don't already have on hand, plus set aside a good time for you to tackle your first project.

Here's to beautiful—and delicious—craft projects straight from the kitchen.

Have fun!

Charity

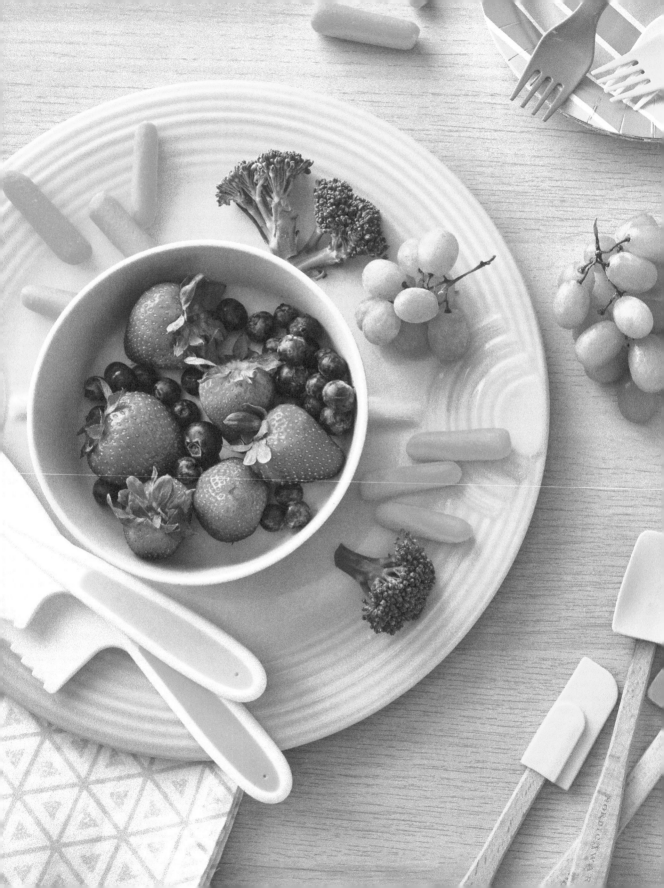

PART 1

Getting Ready

Rules of the Kitchen

The kitchen is such a fun space, especially with all these tasty treats, but using knives, stoves, and other cooking tools can be dangerous. Follow these guidelines to stay safe.

Adult supervision: Watch for the ask an adult warnings in this book. That means stop! You will need help from a grown-up to cut an ingredient, take a pan out of the oven, or do another step that could be dangerous for kids.

Clean hands: Give them a good scrub before you get started! Use warm water with plenty of soap and be sure to rub each part of your hands and fingers together before rinsing, for at least 20 seconds.

Clean work area: Before you start crafting, clear a space on your counter. Then use a clean cloth to wipe down the surface.

Clean ingredients: Using fresh fruit or veggies? Give them a nice rinse under cool water before adding them to your recipe.

Safe food handling: Most of the ingredients in this book are already cooked, but don't forget to put things like cheese, eggs, and milk back in the refrigerator. Leaving them out for more than 3 hours can promote bacteria growth.

Clean as you go: If you haven't noticed, it's important to have a clean kitchen! Keep a clean cloth on hand to wipe up any spills (and your hands). It's also handy to have a garbage bowl to put wrappers and scraps into, rather than walking across the kitchen to the garbage again and again.

Cooking and Crafting Tools

Having the right equipment makes crafting easy and fun. But the good news is that if you don't have everything here, there's no need to worry! There are plenty of ways to substitute household items for specialty tools. Here are some items you might need to make these edible crafts:

Tools and utensils

Cutting board, colander, grater, spoons, mixing bowls, pastry brush, scissors, knives (paring and bread knives for grown-ups, kid-safe knives for kids), spatulas, measuring cups and spoons, cookie cutters, ice pop molds, wooden craft sticks, straws, parchment paper, bamboo skewers, toothpicks

Cookware and bakeware

Baking sheets, baking pans, saucepans, skillet

Appliances

Electric mixer (handheld or stand), food processor (optional), microwave oven

Crafty Cooking Essentials

Are you ready to get crafty? Just follow these simple steps to make your projects as successful—and delicious—as possible:

1. **Read the recipe.** Look through the ingredient list and read all the instructions before you start. That gives you an idea of what you'll be doing and when.

2. **Check that you have all the ingredients and tools.** Nothing's worse than thinking you have all the required ingredients only to find out that someone ate the last of the item you need. Check your pantry, refrigerator, and tool area ahead of time and ask a grown-up to buy more of what you need.

3. **Get out all the ingredients and tools.** On the day you're ready to make a food craft, set all your ingredients and equipment on your clean counter. That way you aren't racing around the kitchen trying to find something in the middle of a recipe.

4. **Measure carefully.** Most of the recipes in this book are very adaptable, but do start out with the measurements given. That's what worked best when we made all the recipes at home. If you want to add a little more here or there, that'll be up to you.

5. **Always be safe.** The worst way to end a craft project is in the emergency room! Follow the safety instructions and always ask a grown-up for help when you're not sure.

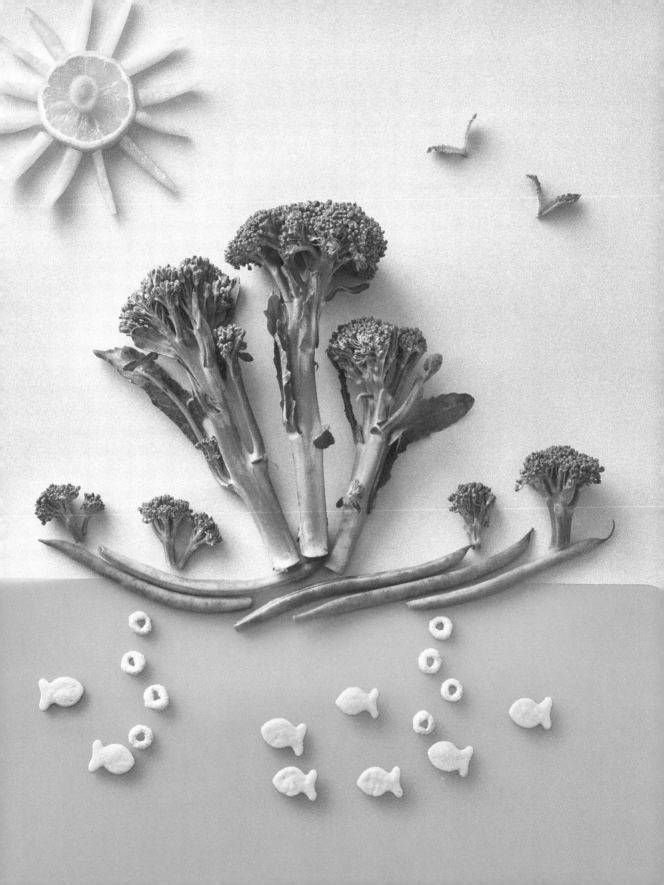

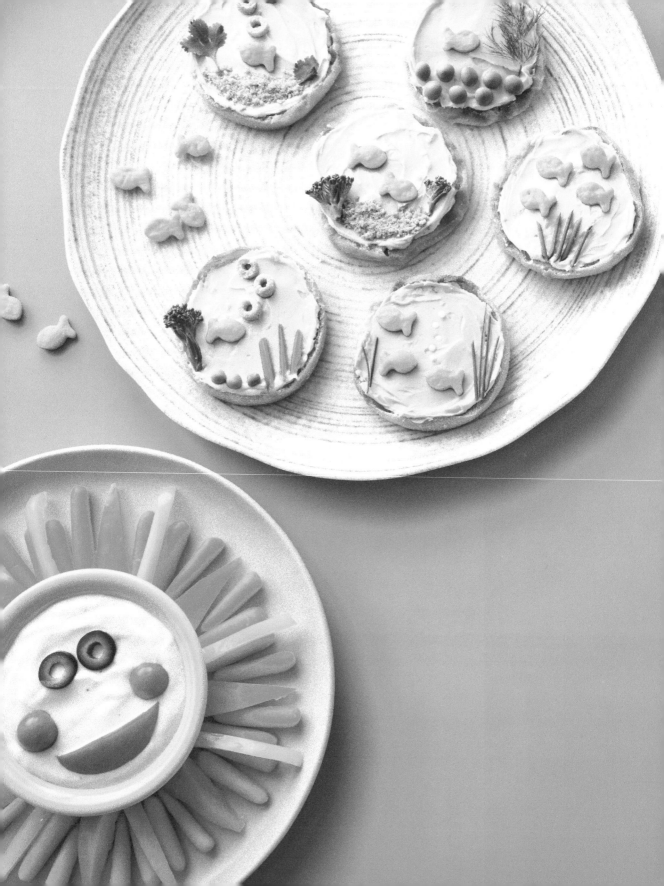

⇒ PART 2 ⇐

Fun Food Crafts

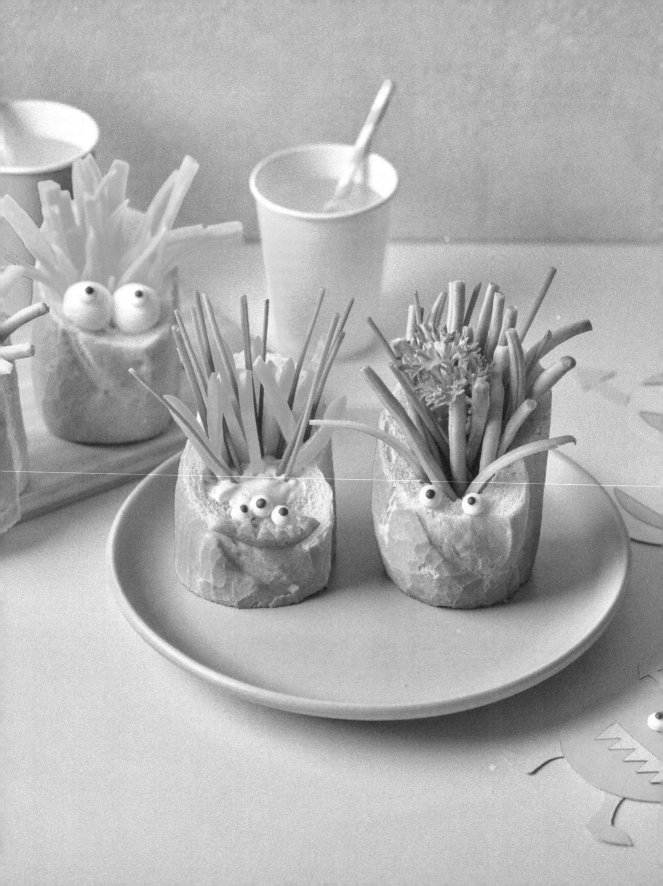

Monster Veggie Cups

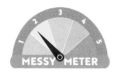

EASY

Nut-Free Vegetarian

Prep time: 15 minutes
Yield: 6 to 8 monsters

Ingredients

1 French baguette

½ cup Greek yogurt

¼ cup ranch dressing

Veggie sticks, such as
carrots, bell peppers,
cucumbers, green
beans, celery

Herb sprigs, such as
dill, parsley, chives
(optional)

12 to 16 candy eyeballs

Tools/Equipment

Bread knife

Cutting board

Small bowl

Spoon

Who's afraid of a few vegetables? Not these monsters! Once you crunch through all your tasty veggies with dip, you get to eat the cup too!

1. **Make the bread cups.** Ask an adult to help cut the baguette. First trim the ends off the baguette. Next, cut the baguette on an angle to make a section about 4 inches long. Then cut the next 4-inch section straight. Repeat the diagonal and straight cuts until you have sliced the whole baguette into 4-inch pieces with one tall side. Scoop out the bread from the center of each piece of bread on the tall side but leave the flat bottom intact so that the dip doesn't leak out.

2. **Add the dip.** In a small bowl, combine the yogurt and ranch dressing, then stir with a spoon. Spoon some dip into each bread cup.

3. **Fill with veggies.** Stand up as many vegetables as possible in the bread cup, so one end is sitting in the dip and the other pokes out above the cup. Add herbs too, if you like.

→

4. **Add the eyes.** Using a little bit of dip, "glue" the eyeballs to the front of your bread cup.

TOP TIPS

▶ Did you take out too much bread from the bottom of your bread cups? Just use your finger to poke some back in.

▶ The yogurt helps thicken the ranch dressing and makes a better consistency for this project.

▶ Want a gluten-free option? Use a cucumber instead of a baguette!

DID YOU KNOW?

▶ Vegetables are grown from seeds.

▶ Most vegetables need warm weather to grow. But some vegetables, like spinach, lettuce, carrots, and turnips, can grow in cold weather.

▶ Ranch dressing is the most popular salad dressing flavor in America, with Italian running a distant second.

JUST FOR LAUGHS
What kind of flower doesn't go in a vase?
Cauliflower!

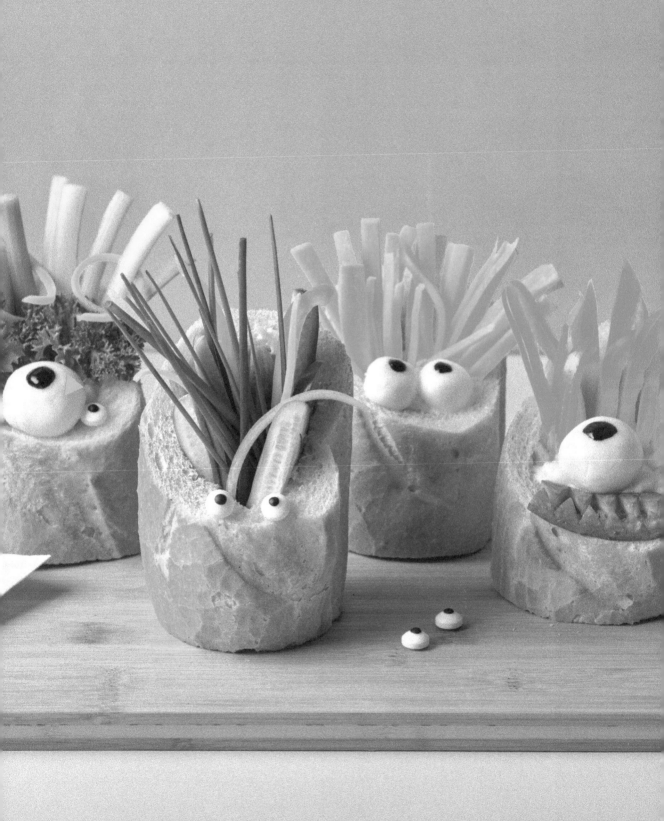

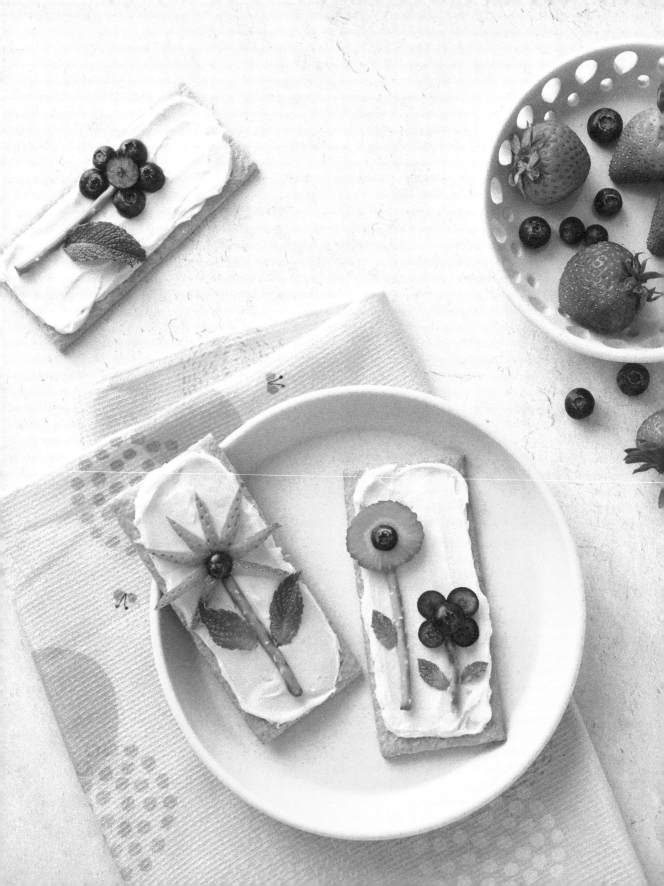

Flower Garden Graham Crackers

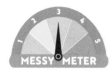

EASY

Nut-Free Vegetarian

Prep time: 15 minutes
Yield: 4 crackers

Ingredients

½ cup vanilla or cream cheese frosting

4 graham crackers

4 pretzel sticks

2 cups fresh berries (strawberries, blueberries, raspberries) or sliced melon (cantaloupe, honeydew)

Fresh mint or parsley leaves

Tools/Equipment

Kid-safe knife

What's sweeter than a flower garden? One made of fruit and frosting! These tasty treats are perfect for an after-school visit with friends. Everyone can make their own, with their favorite designs and combinations of fruit. Then it's time to enjoy! These treats are best when you eat them right away.

When you're all finished, share your creations! Take a photo and use hashtag #LittleFoodies on social media.

1. **Spread the frosting.** Use a kid-safe knife to spread a thick layer of frosting on each graham cracker. This is the base that your decorations will stick to.

2. **Create fruit flowers.** Think about how you want your garden to look. Arrange berries or slices of fruit in any combination to make flowers.

3. **Add a pretzel stem.** Place 1 pretzel stick in the middle of the graham cracker, running top to bottom. This will be the stem.

4. **Add herbs for leaves.** Finish with mint or parsley leaves.

→

TOP TIPS

▶ Want to use chocolate or strawberry frosting? Please do! Use any flavor (or color) you like.

▶ Make your flower garden look more realistic by using fresh chives as the stem and add crumbled chocolate cookies such as Oreos to the base, like dirt!

▶ Nine graham crackers come in each sleeve, so you might want to double up on ingredients (and save room in your tummies) to use them all.

 DID YOU KNOW?

▶ Graham crackers were invented by Sylvester Graham. He was a minister who created the recipe in 1829.

▶ Strawberries usually have a bright red color, but they can also come in pinkish and white colors.

▶ Blueberries are native to North America and come in many varieties. In general, you'll find "highbush" blueberries at the grocery store and "lowbush" berries (which are smaller and sweeter) made into syrups or muffin mixes.

▶ Until the 1930s, pretzels were handmade, and the average worker could twist 40 a minute.

JUST FOR LAUGHS
What did the big flower say to the little one? *Move over, bud!*
What did the strawberry say when she got a gift? *Thank you berry much!*

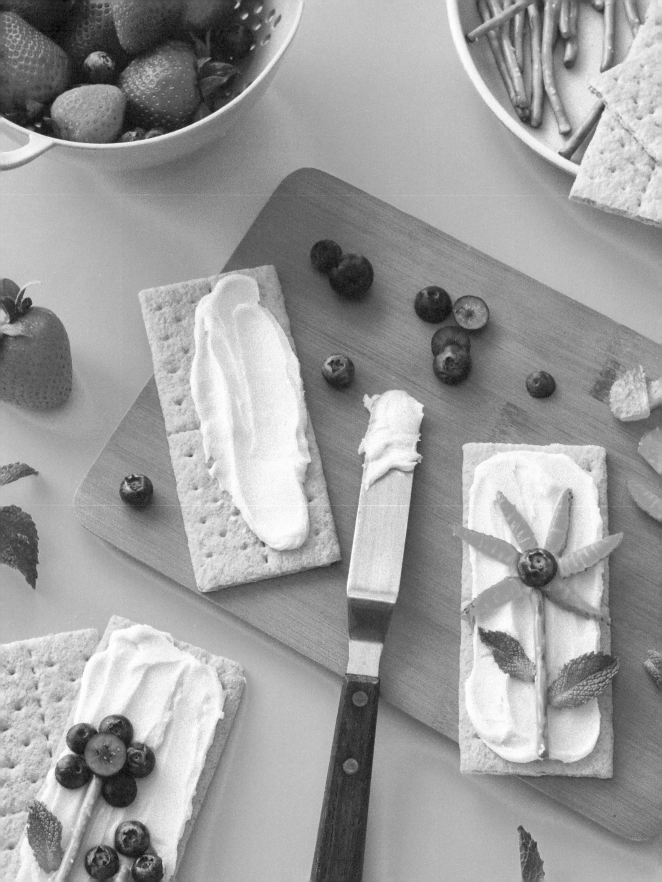

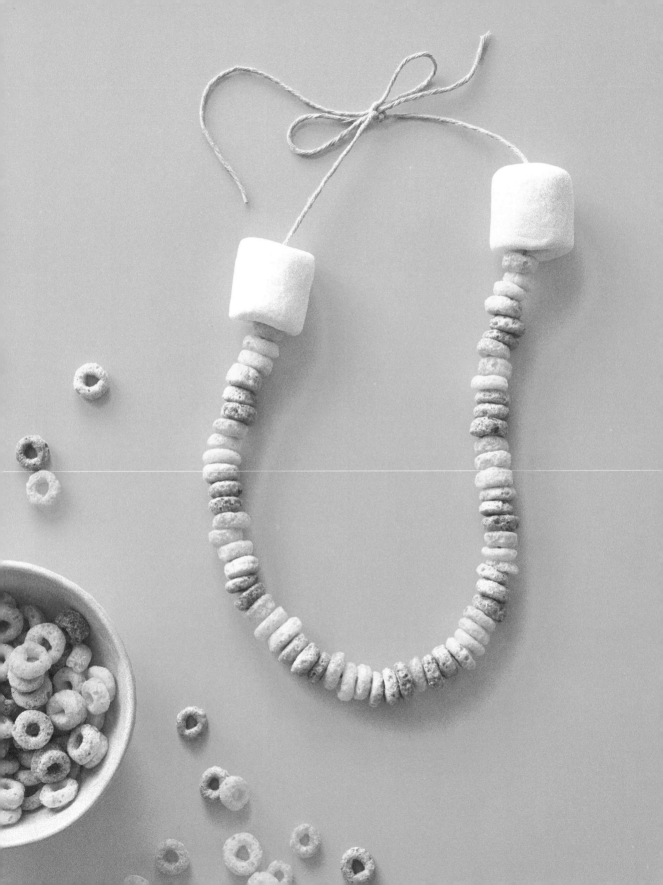

Over the Rainbow Cereal Necklaces

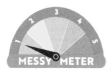

MEDIUM

Dairy-Free Nut-Free

Prep time: 20 minutes
Yield: 6 to 8 necklaces

Ingredients

Marshmallows
(16-ounce bag)

Colored O-shaped
cereal, such as Froot
Loops (10-ounce box)

Tools/Equipment

String (about 2½ feet
for each necklace)

Scissors

Bowls or trays
(1 for each person)

Plastic straws

Make your own colorful fashion statement that doubles as a snack! Our kids love making these necklaces before going on a hike, then munching on the trail. Necklaces are also a fun party project that friends can take home as a parting gift. For maximum fun and minimal mess, let each kid have a tray or baking sheet to use as their personal work space.

When you're all finished, share your creations! Take a photo and use hashtag #LittleFoodies on social media.

1. **Cut the string.** Start by measuring how long you want your necklace to be. Loop the string around your shoulders to estimate the length, leaving enough room for tying a knot. Then cut the string with scissors.

2. **Make a marshmallow hole.** Use a straw to pierce a marshmallow through the center. Push the straw through until some of it comes out the other side.

3. **Thread the marshmallow.** With the straw still inside the marshmallow, slide your string through the straw like you're →

pushing it through a tunnel. Remove the straw, leaving the marshmallow on the string.

4. **Make a rainbow.** Thread your cereal O's onto the string but don't fill the entire length. Stop after about 25 pieces and hold the necklace up to your chest to measure. Finish if you like how it looks, or add more O's, leaving enough room for another marshmallow "cloud" and to tie the string too.

5. **Add another marshmallow.** Repeat steps 2 and 3 so that you have marshmallow "clouds" on either side of the cereal rainbow.

6. **Tie the string.** Tie the ends of the string together and make a knot. Slip your necklace over your head and eat it while you wear it!

 ## DID YOU KNOW?

▶ Marshmallows date all the way back to ancient Egypt. Originally they were made with a plant in the mallow family that grows in marshes. That's why they're called marshmallows!

▶ More than half of all marshmallows purchased in the United States are toasted over a fire.

▶ The first book to share a recipe for s'mores, combining chocolate bars, graham crackers, and toasted marshmallows, was *The Girl Scout Handbook* in 1927.

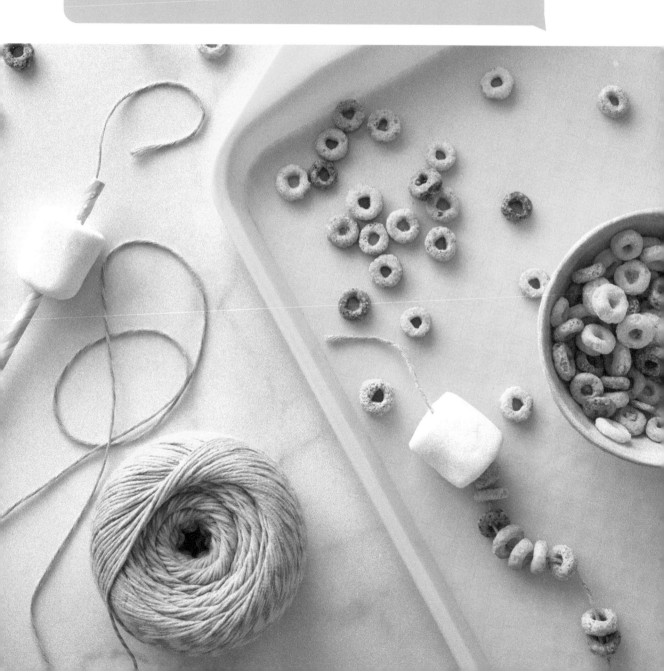

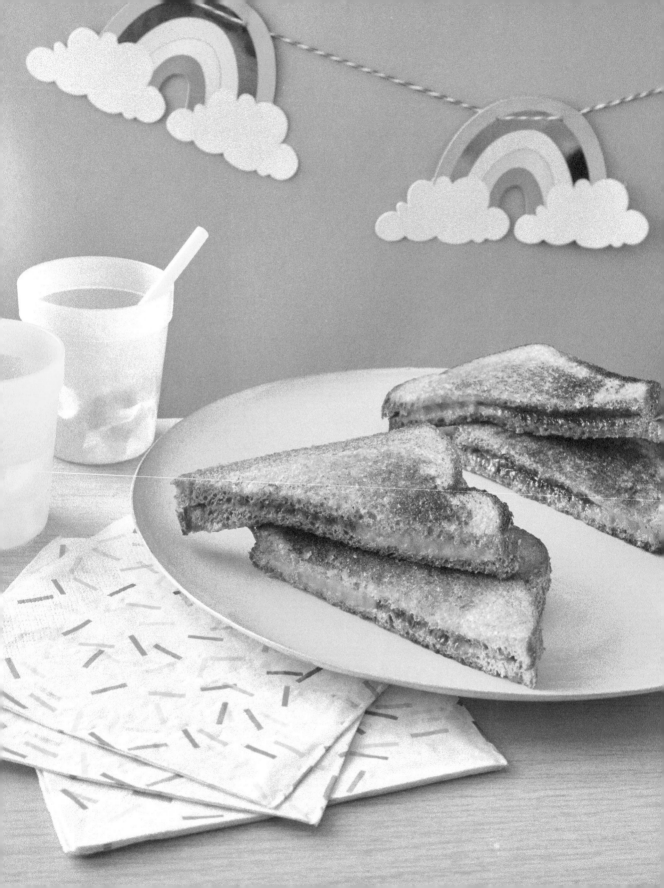

Unicorn Grilled Cheese

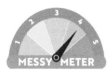

HARD

Nut-Free Vegetarian

Prep time: 15 minutes
Cook time: 5 minutes
Yield: 4 sandwiches

Ingredients

2 cups shredded white cheddar cheese

Food coloring in 4 colors

8 slices sandwich bread

Butter or mayonnaise

Tools/Equipment

4 small bowls

4 forks

Kid-safe knife

4 plates

Skillet

Flipping spatula

This isn't your average everyday grilled cheese! The surprise comes when you cut into this beautiful sandwich, unleashing a full rainbow of ooey-gooey cheesy goodness fit for a unicorn.

1. **Color the cheese.** Divide the cheese evenly among the 4 bowls. Add 3 to 6 drops of food coloring to each bowl, using a different color for each. Use the forks to fluff the cheese, stirring until each piece is at least partly coated with color. (Don't worry! When the cheese melts, the colors will even out.)

2. **Coat the outside of your bread.** Use a kid-safe knife to spread one side of each piece of bread with either butter or my secret ingredient, mayonnaise! This helps the bread get golden brown.

3. **Assemble the rainbow.** To make each sandwich, place 1 piece of bread on a plate with the butter/mayonnaise side down. Add rows of colored cheese starting at the top of the bread. Make a strip →

of red, then yellow after that, followed by green, and blue (or whatever colors you're using). Place the second piece of bread on top, with the butter/mayonnaise side up.

4. **Cook the sandwich.** Ask an adult to heat a skillet on the stove over low heat. Carefully transfer each sandwich to the skillet. Grill the first side until the edges of the bread are golden brown and the cheese starts to melt. Use a spatula to carefully flip and grill the other side for another couple of minutes, until browned.

5. **Reveal the rainbow.** Ask an adult to cut the sandwiches in the middle so you can see the cheesy colors inside.

 ## TOP TIPS

▶ If the bread is browning too quickly without the cheese melting completely, turn the burner off and let the cheese melt with the remaining heat.

▶ For a fun variation, substitute small tortillas for bread and make a unicorn quesadilla!

▶ Get extra fancy and use a large cookie cutter to cut the bread into a fun shape, like a heart or star, before starting.

> **JUST FOR LAUGHS**
> What do you call sad cheese? *Blue cheese!*

▶ The ancient Romans are thought to be the first people to make sandwiches from cooked bread and cheese.

▶ In Switzerland, people often toast the bread and melt the cheese separately before combining them together.

▶ In France, a grilled ham and cheese sandwich, called a *croque monsieur*, is very popular—and very delicious!

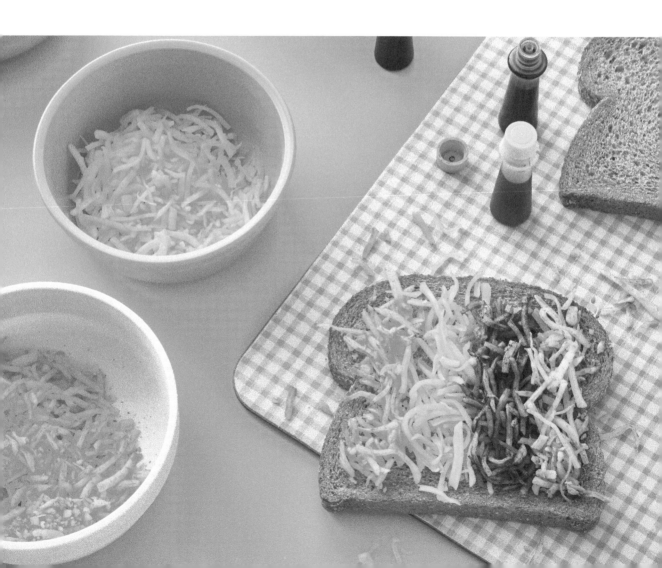

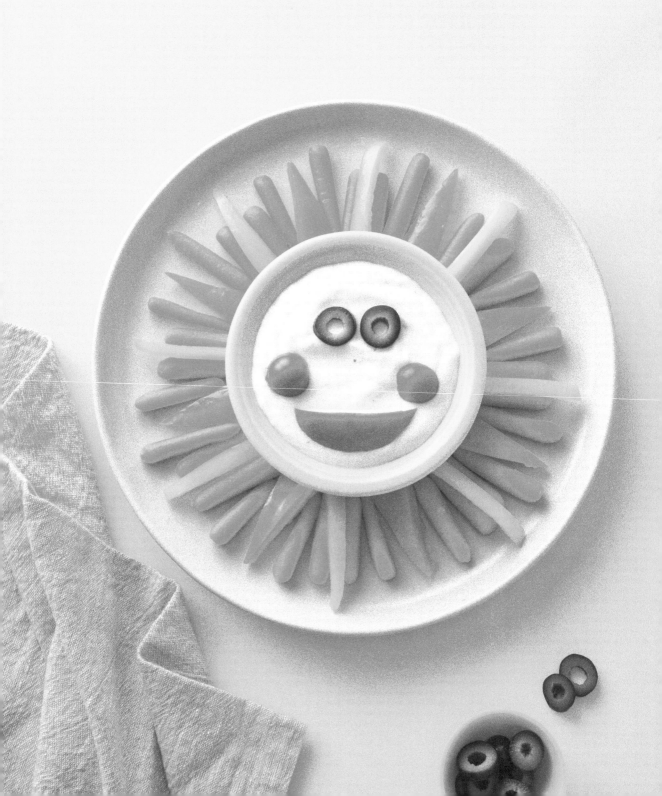

Sunshine Fun Dip with Crunchy Veggies

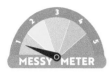

EASY

Nut-Free
Gluten-Free
Vegetarian

Prep time: 15 minutes
Yield: 4 servings

Ingredients

1 cup Greek yogurt

¼ cup blue cheese or ranch dressing

1 yellow bell pepper, seeded and cut into strips

1 orange bell pepper, seeded and cut into strips

1 cup baby carrots

2 black olive slices

1 red apple slice

1 cherry tomato, cut in half

Tools/Equipment

Small bowl

Spoon

Plate

Here's your chance to dazzle a crowd with the sunniest, funniest face a veggie plate ever saw. Use blue cheese or ranch dressing to flavor the Greek yogurt dip, but watch out—the result is so yummy (and even nutritious) that everyone will want to double-dip!

1. **Make the dip.** Combine the yogurt and dressing in a small bowl and stir until mixed well. Place the bowl in the center of a plate.

2. **Arrange the veggies.** Arrange the pepper strips and carrots in a circle around the bowl of dip so that the ends are facing out.

3. **Add the face.** Put the olive slices in the middle to act as eyes. Add the apple slice underneath for the smile. For a finishing touch, add the cherry tomato halves as cheeks.

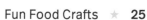

DID YOU KNOW?

▶ Since bell peppers have seeds and come from flowering plants, they are actually fruits, not vegetables. This is true for many foods we think of as vegetables!

▶ Bell peppers are packed with vitamin C. Eating one large red pepper gives you 300 percent of the vitamin C you need in a day, three times more than an orange!

▶ Carrots are usually orange, but they come in many other colors too, including purple, red, yellow, and white.

▶ Carrots are made of about 88 percent water and bell peppers are even more, at 92 percent.

▶ In the United States, India, Canada, and Malaysia, we say bell peppers. But in Australia and New Zealand they're called cap-sicums. In England, they're just called peppers. And in Japan? They say papurika.

▶ The green leafy part of a carrot is edible too!

JUST FOR LAUGHS

How do you know carrots are good for your eyes? *You never see rabbits wearing glasses.*

Why did the sun go to school? *To get brighter!*

What did one snowman say to the other one? *Does it smell like carrots out here to you?*

EXTRA CRAFTY

Instead of a sun, make this a lion! Just change the mouth: Skip the apple slice and use a tube of black writing frosting to draw a lion's mouth like a letter W. Draw a picture of what you want to try next time in the space below.

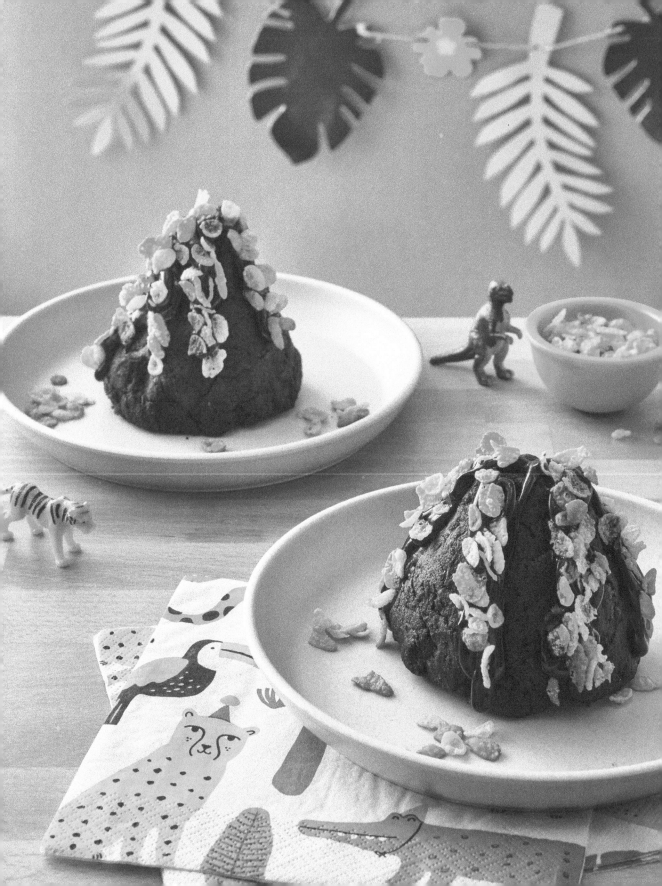

Fiery Flowing Volcano Cakes

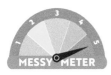

HARD

Nut-Free Vegetarian

Prep time: 20 minutes, plus cooling time
Cook time: 35 minutes
Yield: 4 to 8 cakes

Ingredients

Nonstick cooking spray

1 box chocolate cake mix (12 to 15 ounces), plus required oil and eggs

1 tub (1 pound) chocolate frosting

Red, orange, and yellow cereal, such as Fruity Pebbles

Tools/Equipment

9 x 13-inch baking pan

Electric mixer (handheld or stand)

Large bowl

Silicone spatula

Large spoon

Chocolate flavor is positively overflowing with these mini volcano cakes! One cake mix makes enough for four large volcanos, or you can divide the mixture into as many as eight smaller volcanoes.

1. **Bake the cake.** Preheat the oven to the temperature called for on the cake mix box. Coat a 9 x 13-inch baking pan with nonstick spray. Ask an adult to help you use an electric mixer to mix the cake ingredients in a large bowl according to the instructions. Pour the batter into the prepared pan, carefully put the pan in the oven, and bake according to the instructions until the cake is cooked through and the sides pull away from the pan, usually 30 to 35 minutes. Ask an adult to help you remove the pan from the oven and set it aside to cool fully. (Note: This step can be done up to 3 days ahead of time; store the cake in an air-tight container at room temperature.)

2. **Crumble the cake.** Find a second large bowl, then dump the cooled cake into it. Use your hands to crumble the whole cake.

→

Tools/Equipment
continued

4 plates

Small microwave-safe bowl

3. **Add the frosting.** Spoon half of the frosting from the tub into the bowl. Use your hands to combine the frosting and crumbled cake until you can squeeze the cake mixture into balls in your hands.

4. **Sculpt the volcanos.** Divide the cake mixture into 4 equal sections and place 1 on each plate. Mold the cake with your hands into the shape of a volcano.

5. **Add the lava.** Put the remaining chocolate frosting in a microwave-safe bowl. Ask an adult to help heat the frosting until it's pourable, in bursts of 10 seconds, stirring in between. Pour the frosting on the top edges of each volcano. Stick red, orange, and yellow pieces of cereal onto the frosting.

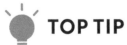 **TOP TIP**

▶ Sort out the cereal by color ahead of time.

DID YOU KNOW?

- Volcanoes are classified in three ways: active, dormant, or extinct. "Active" means there's regular activity in the volcano. "Dormant" volcanoes are volcanoes that are currently quiet. "Extinct" volcanoes haven't erupted in so long that they're unlikely to ever erupt again. Right now, there are about 1,900 active volcanoes on Earth.

- Magma is hot liquid rock inside a volcano. Once it leaves the volcano, it's referred to as lava.

- Other planets and moons have volcanoes, too! The largest volcano in our solar system is Olympus Mons, found on Mars.

JUST FOR LAUGHS
What did one volcano say to the other?
I lava you.

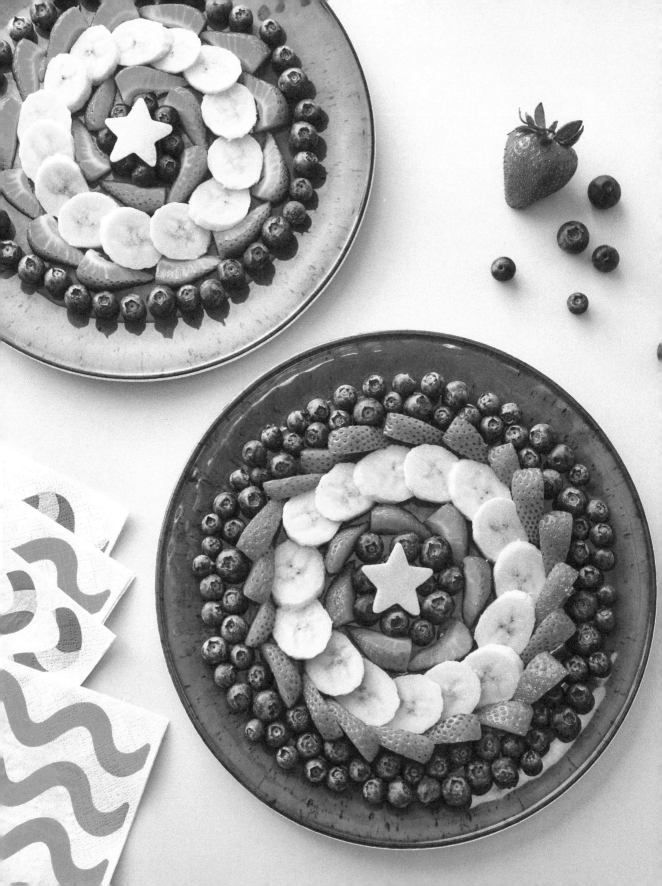

Captain America's Colorful Fruit Plate

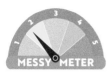

EASY

Gluten-Free
Nut-Free
Vegetarian

Prep time: 15 minutes
Yield: 4 fruit plates

Ingredients

2 pints blueberries

4 slices white cheddar cheese

2 pints strawberries, cut into quarters or eighths

2 bananas

Tools/Equipment

4 plates or
1 large platter

Star-shaped
cookie cutter

Cutting board

Kid-safe knife

What do you call a shield made out of strawberries, blueberries, bananas, and cheese? Delicious . . . and perfect for Captain America himself! This sweet snack serves four friends. Make individual fruit plates or ask a grown-up to help you find a large serving platter or cutting board to create one huge shield, before digging in and enjoying together! These fruit shields are best when eaten right away, so plan for enough time to make your plates and snack too. No Avenger ever had it so good.

When you're all finished, share your creations! Take a photo and use hashtag #LittleFoodies on social media.

1. **Make a circle of blueberries.** Arrange a handful of blueberries (about 10) in a circle in the center of each plate.

2. **Cut out the star.** Press a star-shaped cookie cutter into each slice of cheese. Very carefully use your fingers to remove the star from the cutter. Set the star on top of the blueberries. (You can snack on the cheese scraps!)

3. **Make a red ring.** Put a ring of sliced strawberries around the blueberries.

4. **Make a white ring.** Use a kid-safe knife to slice the bananas. Arrange them around the strawberries.

5. **Repeat the red ring.** Add more strawberries around the bananas.

6. **Finish with a blue ring.** Add one more row of blueberries on the outer edge.

DID YOU KNOW?

▶ A single banana is called a finger and a bunch of bananas is called a hand.

▶ Blueberries are full of vitamin C, fiber, and antioxidants. Scientists believe these berries can fight disease, prevent some kinds of cancer, and even build healthy brain function.

▶ Strawberries are the first fruit to ripen each spring.

▶ Ancient Romans thought strawberries could cure bad breath and fainting.

▶ Many types of shields were used in Marvel films: rubber for fight scenes, magnetic when worn by Captain America, and even digitally created shields when he threw them!

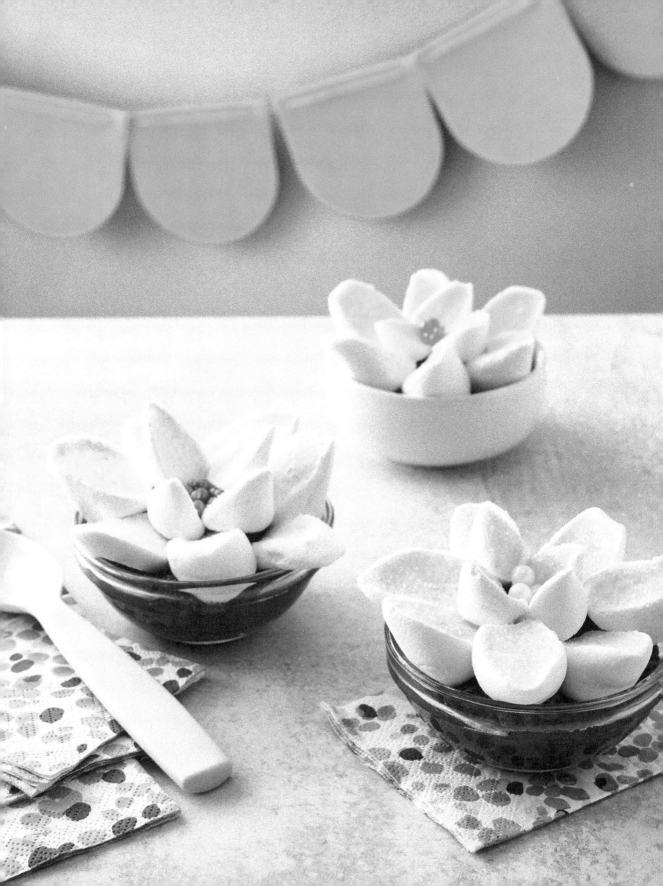

Marshmallow Flower Pudding Pots

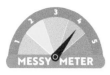

HARD

Nut-Free

Prep time: 20 minutes
Yield: 4 pudding pots

Ingredients

2 cups chocolate pudding (use an instant mix or pre-made pudding cups)

6 to 8 chocolate wafer cookies such as Oreos

Glitter sprinkles (pink, purple, red, or whatever combination you like)

25 to 30 marshmallows

Fresh mint leaves (optional)

Sugar pearls (optional)

Tools/Equipment

4 small bowls

Food processor or zip-top plastic bag and mallet

Mixing bowl

Paring knife

Cutting board

Pretty flowers perched on top of chocolate pots—what could be more fun? Chocolate pudding with crumbled cookies make the "dirt." You add the flowers by cutting marshmallows and dipping them in sparkly sprinkles. Add a finishing touch with fresh mint or colorful sugar pearls and your work is done. These pudding cups are best to eat right after you make them so that the cookies stay fresh.

1. **Fill the pudding pots.** Divide the pudding into 4 bowls, leaving enough room for chocolate crumbles on top.

2. **Add chocolate dirt.** Twist the cookies apart and scrape off the white frosting. Throw the frosting away (or eat!). Ask an adult to help blitz the cookies in a food processor until fine, like sand. (No food processor? Put the cookies in a zip-top plastic bag and gently smash with a mallet or a rolling pin if that's what you have. Make sure you set the bag on a strong surface that won't get damaged, like a cutting board on top of a table.) Add a layer of chocolate crumbles on top of the pudding.

➡

3. **Make the flowers.** Pour the glitter sprinkles in a small bowl. Ask an adult to help cut the marshmallows in half on a diagonal. Dip the cut side of each marshmallow into the sprinkles. These are the flower petals! Arrange them in the shape of flowers on top of the dirt cups with the sprinkle-side up.

4. **Finish off with mint and pearls.** If you're using mint, now is the time to add a couple of leaves on the outer rim of the bowl. If you have sugar pearls, set 1 to 3 in the middle of each flower.

 TOP TIP

▶ This sliced marshmallow technique works for lots of other projects too! See page 45, where you'll learn how to make ears for adorable barnyard animals on a stick.

JUST FOR LAUGHS
What do you call a flower that runs on electricity?
A power plant!

EXTRA CRAFTY

You can create almost any design with this idea! What other colors or shapes could you make? Draw a picture of what you want to try next time in the space below.

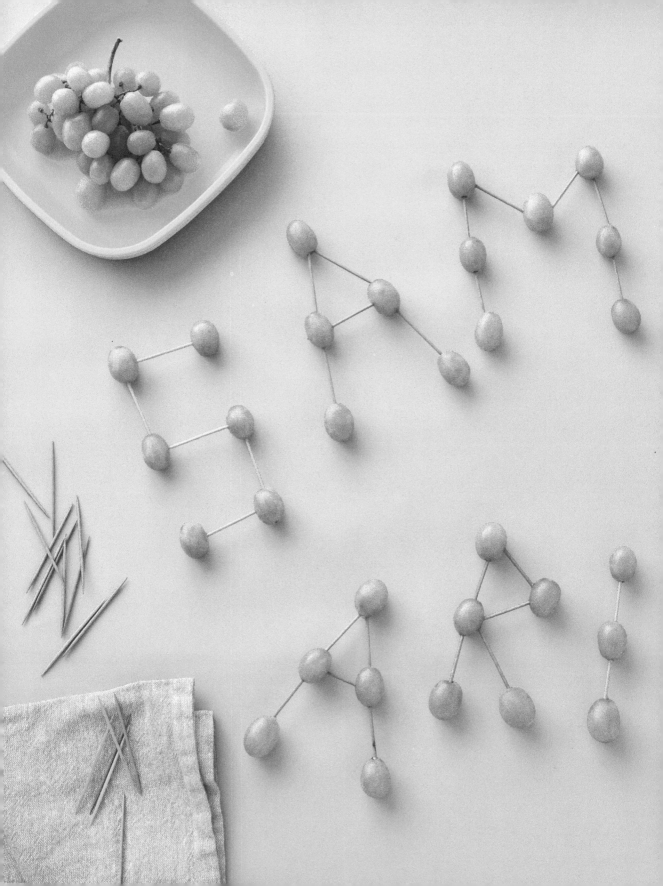

Write Your Name in Grapes

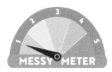

MEDIUM

Dairy-Free
Gluten-Free
Nut-Free
Vegetarian

Prep time: 15 minutes
Yield: 2 or more names

Ingredients

Grapes

Tools/Equipment

Large tray (optional)

Toothpicks

Have you ever dreamed of seeing your name in lights? Or on a billboard? Now you can write your name in jumbo letters, using a simple combination of grapes and toothpicks! Use green or red grapes, or a combination. Spell out your name or initials. Connect each letter or set them side-by-side. Whatever you do, make sure there's plenty of space because your name is about to get big!

When you're all finished, share your creations! Take a photo and use hashtag #LittleFoodies on social media.

1. **Get the grapes ready.** Wash your grapes in the sink. Allow them to dry for a couple of minutes. Pull off the stems and toss any squishy grapes into the compost. If you want, set out a tray to work on.

2. **Piece together the letters.** Find the hole where the stem was on your grapes. This is the best place to stick a toothpick into. Start working to create your name by sliding a toothpick into the hole of

1 grape, then add another grape on the other end. When you need to make a bend, just stick your next toothpick into the grape at an angle. Keep going until you have your name or initials spelled out.

TOP TIP

▶ Pitted olives would also work! Use green or black olives.

DID YOU KNOW?

▶ People have been growing grapes for over 8,000 years, but wild grapes have been around for 65,000 years!

▶ Grapes are actually berries.

▶ Grapes come in many different colors: red, black, green, orange, yellow, blue, and pink.

▶ In the 1600s, toothpicks were made of gold, silver, and ivory, and used over and over. Some even had precious stones set in them!

▶ Toothpicks are considered so handy that you'll always find one included in the tools on a Swiss Army knife.

- More than 90 percent of today's toothpicks are produced in Maine.
- People use toothpicks for lots of creative purposes. A man named Joe King built a model of the Eiffel Tower with 110,000 toothpicks, which reached 23 feet!

JUST FOR LAUGHS

Why did the grape stop in the middle of the road?

He ran out of juice.

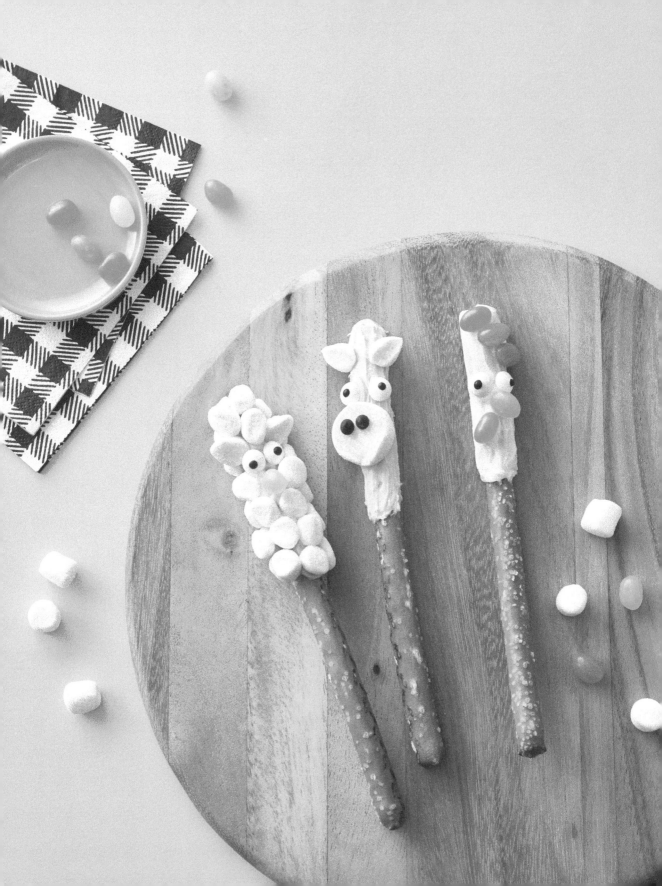

Barnyard Pretzel Stick Snacks

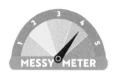

HARD

Nut-Free

Prep time: 15 minutes
Yield: 3 snacks

Ingredients

10 mini marshmallows

2 teaspoons pink sprinkles

½ cup vanilla frosting or white candy melts, liquefied

3 pretzel rods

6 candy eyeballs

Jelly beans: 1 pink, 4 red, 1 orange

¼ cup strawberry frosting or pink candy melts, liquefied, with 1 candy melt reserved

2 mini chocolate chips

Tools/Equipment

Large tray

Parchment paper

Paring knife

Barnyard fun is just minutes away! You and your friends will be making fluffy sheep, pink pigs, and roosters ready to crow. They're not only adorable, though—you'll love the tasty combination of sweet, salty, crunchy, and chewy. These tasty treats are best when you eat them soon after creating them, so give yourself enough time to make and enjoy.

FOR THE SHEEP

1. **Cut the mini marshmallows.** Ask an adult to cut 1 mini marshmallow in half on the diagonal (for the ears) and 8 mini marshmallows in half through the middle (for the fleece).

2. **Make the ears.** Pour a teaspoon of pink sprinkles into a small bowl. Dip the cut side of the diagonally sliced marshmallows into the pink sprinkles.

3. **Coat the pretzel rod.** Use a kid-safe knife to spread vanilla frosting (or liquefied white candy melts) to cover the top half of 1 pretzel rod.

Tools/Equipment

continued

Cutting board

Small bowls

Kid-safe knife

4. **Assemble the sheep.** Line the pretzel stick with cut marshmallows, starting with the back so that it won't stick when you put it down. Attach 2 eyeballs in the middle of the front of the pretzel. Put a pink jelly bean under the eyes as a nose. Set the marshmallow ears off to the sides and fill in the rest of the pretzel with more cut marshmallows.

FOR THE PIG

5. **Make the ears.** Ask an adult to cut 1 mini marshmallow in half on the diagonal. Pour a teaspoon of pink sprinkles into a small bowl (or reuse the same bowl from the sheep). Dip the cut side of the diagonally sliced marshmallows into the pink sprinkles.

6. **Coat the pretzel rod.** Use a kid-safe knife to spread strawberry frosting (or liquefied pink candy melts) to cover the top half of 1 pretzel rod.

7. **Assemble the pig.** Stick on 2 eyeballs, then place the marsh-mallow ears above them. Place 1 pink candy melt right below the eyes. Use a little of the melted candy as glue to attach 2 mini chocolate chips as the snout.

FOR THE ROOSTER

8. **Coat the pretzel rod.** Use a kid-safe knife to spread vanilla frosting (or liquefied white candy melts) to cover the top half of 1 pretzel rod.

9. **Assemble the rooster.** Stick 3 red jelly beans at the top of the pretzel rod in a slight curve. Add 2 eyeballs. Place 1 slightly crooked orange jelly bean under the eyes and 1 more red jelly bean under it, at the other angle.

 TOP TIP

▶ Candy melts dry into a stiffer, firmer, and less sticky final prod-uct, but frosting is a little simpler to use because you don't have to melt it. If you choose strawberry frosting instead of candy melts for the pig, make sure you have some other type of pink candy to use for the snout.

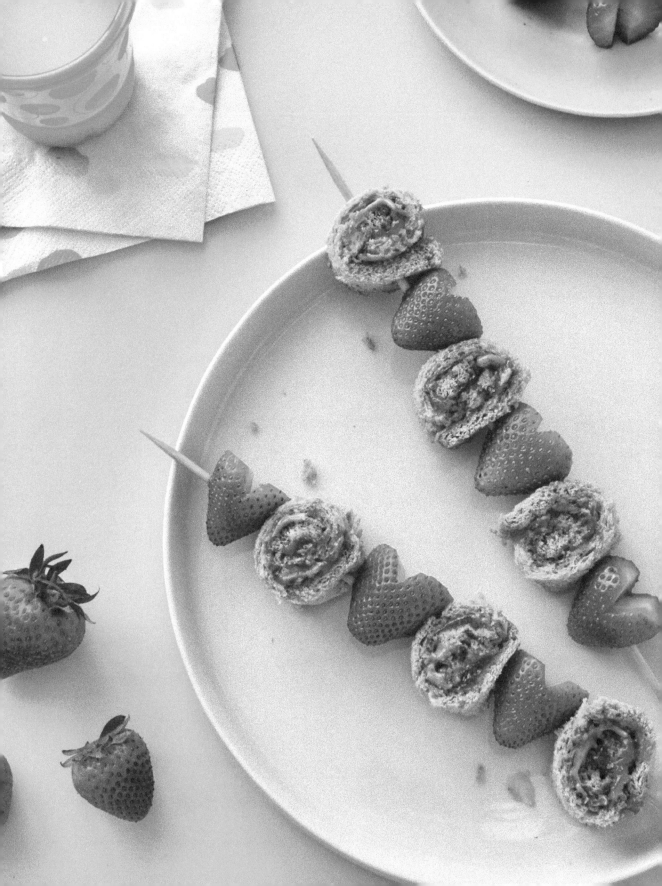

Pinwheel PB&J on a Stick

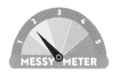

MEDIUM

Dairy-Free
Vegetarian

Prep time: 15 minutes
Yield: 2 skewers

Ingredients

4 to 6 strawberries

2 slices soft
sandwich bread

2 tablespoons
peanut butter

2 teaspoons
strawberry jam

Tools/Equipment

Paring knife

Cutting board

Rolling pin

Kid-safe knife

Bread knife

2 skewers

What's tastier than a peanut butter and jelly sandwich? Sushi-style sandwiches layered with fresh berries on a skewer! Whether crunchy or smooth peanut butter or other nut butter, whole-wheat bread or white, jam flavored with strawberries, raspberries, or blackberries—all the choices are up to you. This recipe makes enough for two skewers, but once you purchase the supplies, you'll have enough to make these treats with a group of friends. These treats are best eaten soon after making.

1. **Cut the strawberries.** Ask an adult to help cut the tops off each strawberry in a V-shape, removing the stems and hulls to create a heart.

2. **Roll out the bread.** Use a rolling pin to roll out each piece of bread until it is smooth and flat.

3. **Coat with peanut butter.** Use a kid-safe knife to spread peanut butter all over the flattened bread slices.

4. **Coat with jam.** Add a very thin layer of jam on top of the peanut butter.

5. **Roll up.** Use your fingers to tightly roll up each piece of bread into a long roll.

6. **Slice.** Ask an adult to help slice each roll-up into bite-size pieces.

7. **Assemble.** Thread alternating pieces of roll-ups and strawberries onto each skewer.

DID YOU KNOW?

▶ Bread, in all its different forms, is the most common food in the world.

▶ People have called money "dough" or "bread" for over a hundred years. It comes from having enough money to buy food!

▶ It takes about 540 peanuts to make a 12-ounce jar of peanut butter.

▶ The world's largest peanut butter factory makes over 250,000 jars of peanut butter every day.

▶ Peanut butter and jelly sandwiches were packed as rations for soldiers in World War II, and when they came home, soldiers made the new sandwich popular for everyone.

▶ Of the top 10 candy bars sold, 4 have either peanuts or peanut butter in them.

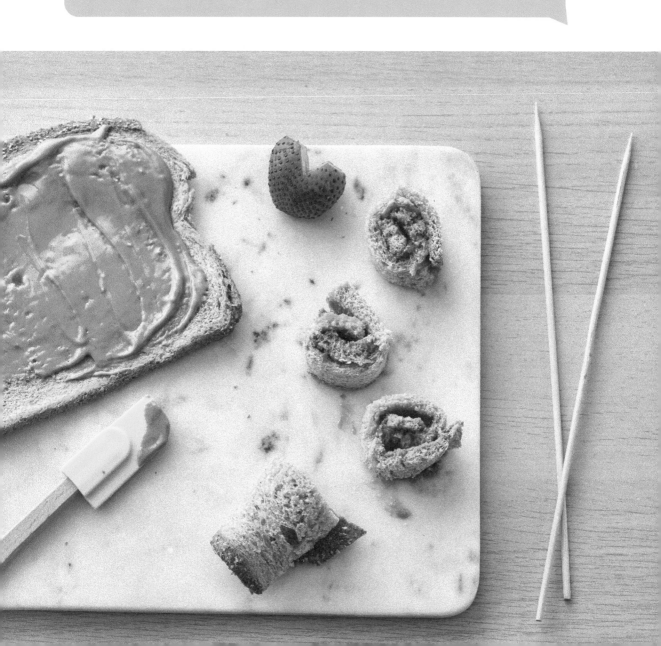

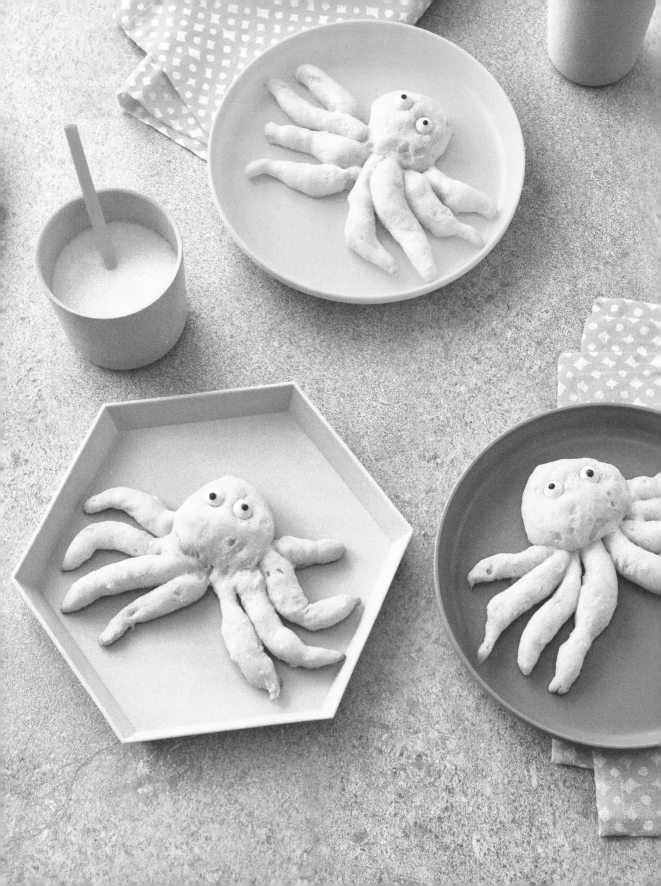

Olly, Olly Octopus Biscuits

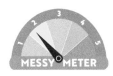

MEDIUM

Nut-Free Vegetarian

Prep time: 5 minutes
Cook time: 15 minutes
Yield: 6 octopus biscuits

Ingredients

1 tube biscuit dough

12 candy eyeballs

Tools/Equipment

2 baking sheets

Parchment paper

Paring knife

Cutting board

Coming straight from the deepest depths of the ocean . . . all the way to your plate! These octopus biscuits are excellent when dipped in a little melted butter, one long arm at a time.

1. **Get ready to bake.** Preheat the oven to 350°F. Line 2 baking sheets with parchment paper.

2. **Cut the dough.** Ask an adult to help cut each biscuit into 4 wedges. Set 1 wedge aside, for the head. Cut a second wedge into 2 pieces, for the longest arms. Cut the last 2 wedges into 3 pieces each, for the 6 remaining legs.

3. **Shape the octopus.** Use your hands to roll the largest wedge of dough into a ball for the head. Then roll the other wedges between your hand and a clean surface until they look like snakes. Place the ball on the parchment-lined baking sheet. Arrange the long legs under the ball so that they connect at the top, branching out and curling up at the bottoms, then add the remaining legs between them. Gently press down on the ball to form a head, making sure to cover the tips of the legs.

4. **Bake.** Carefully place the baking sheets in the oven and bake for 10 minutes. Ask an adult to help remove the sheet from the oven. Carefully press 2 candy eyeballs onto each head. Ask an adult to put the sheet back in the oven and bake for another 2 minutes, then remove from the oven. Let cool for a bit before digging in!

 ## DID YOU KNOW?

▶ Octopuses don't have a skeleton, which means they can squeeze into tight spaces.

▶ An octopus has a hard beak, like a bird, to break into and eat prey like crabs and shellfish.

▶ Octopuses have three hearts.

JUST FOR LAUGHS

What sea creatures say hello sixteen times?
Two octopuses shaking hands.

What do you call an octopus in a band? *A rock-topus!*

EXTRA CRAFTY

What else could you make with biscuit dough? Draw an idea to try in the space below!

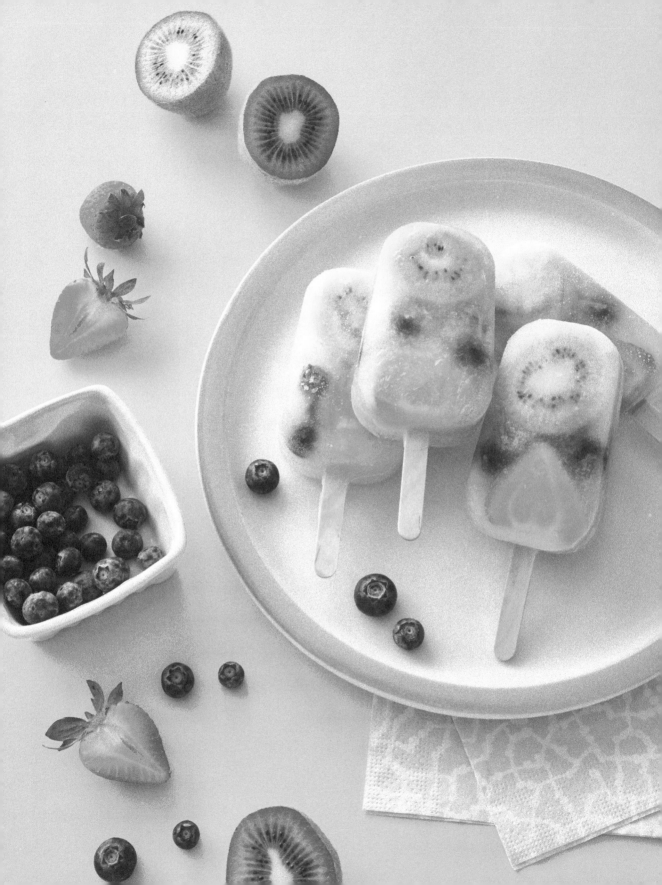

Fresh & Fruity Ice Pops

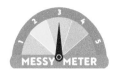

MEDIUM

Dairy-Free
Gluten-Free
Nut-Free
Vegetarian

Prep time: 15 minutes, plus 4 hours to freeze
Yield: 10 ice pops

Ingredients

6 to 8 kiwis

2 pints strawberries

½ pint blueberries

Lemonade

Tools/Equipment

Paring knife

Cutting board

10 ice pop molds

Wooden craft sticks
(if your molds don't
include sticks)

There's nothing like biting into a piece of fresh fruit on a hot day—unless it's a frozen ice pop packed with colorful fruit! You'll want to make them ahead of time since they take a few hours to freeze. Trust me, they're worth the wait!

1. **Slice the big fruit.** Ask an adult to help peel the kiwi and cut off the stems and hulls from the strawberries, then slice both.

2. **Fill the ice pop molds.** Starting with the biggest pieces of fruit, fill each mold with as much fruit as you can fit. Really push the fruit down to fit as much as you can.

3. **Pour in the lemonade.** Pour a little lemonade into each ice pop mold, but not to the top—leave about ½ inch for the stick. Go slowly! You won't need much lemonade.

4. **Add the sticks.** Finish by inserting the wooden sticks, or the sticks that came with your ice pop molds.

5. **Freeze.** Carefully transfer the ice pop molds to the freezer and freeze for at least 4 hours.

 TOP TIPS

▶ To make it easier to fit more fruit in each ice pop, arrange the kiwi and strawberry slices along the edges.

▶ Switch up the flavors! Use sliced fruit of any kind, like peaches and pineapples. Even frozen fruit works great since it's already peeled and sliced.

▶ Go fancy! Puree your choice of fruit in a blender, then fill your ice pop molds and put them in the freezer. When they come out, lay the ice pops on a baking sheet and add chocolate sauce and sprinkles on top, then refreeze. Carefully flip them over, add more chocolate sauce and sprinkles, and refreeze again.

DID YOU KNOW?

▶ Kiwi fruit grows on a vine!

▶ Popsicles were originally marketed as "a frozen drink on a stick."

▶ Popsicles that come with two sticks were invented during the Great Depression so that two children could share an ice pop for only a nickel.

▶ Popsicle sticks are made from birch trees.

JUST FOR LAUGHS
Why do ice pops always get invited to parties?
Because they're cool.

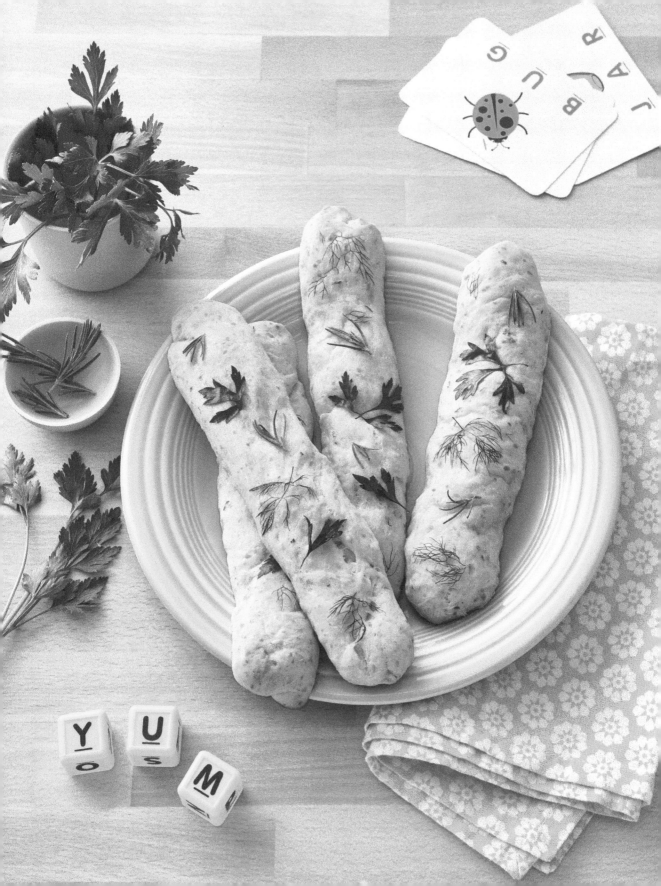

Breadstick Nature Art

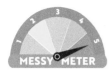

HARD

Nut-Free

Vegetarian

Prep time: 45 minutes, plus 45 minutes to rise
Cook time: 10 minutes
Yield: 12 breadsticks

Ingredients

Nonstick cooking spray

3 cups all-purpose flour, divided, plus ¼ cup for dusting

¼ cup sugar

1 packet (2¼ teaspoons) active dry yeast

1 cup warm water

1 teaspoon salt

4 tablespoons unsalted butter, melted

½ cup shredded Parmesan cheese

1 tablespoon Italian seasoning

Bursting with cheesy flavor and with all the softness of your favorite white bread, these breadsticks are a blank canvas, just waiting for you to show your creative side. This bread needs to rise for 45 minutes, so you'll have time to play in between steps.

1. **Make the dough.** Coat a large bowl with nonstick spray and set aside. Combine 1 cup of flour plus all the sugar and yeast in another large bowl. Add the warm water. (Tip: It should be about the temperature of your bath water.) Set on a warm counter for 10 minutes. When the yeast mixture looks puffy, add another 1 cup of flour, plus the salt and melted butter and stir to combine. Add the remaining 1 cup of flour, Parmesan cheese, and Italian seasoning and stir again to combine well.

2. **Knead the dough.** Scatter the ¼ cup of extra flour on a cutting board or clean countertop, then put the dough on top. The dough will be very sticky! Knead the

Ingredients

continued

Fresh herb sprigs and leaves, such as dill, rosemary, chives, oregano, or parsley

Add-ons, such as chopped olives and bell peppers (optional)

Olive oil

Tools/Equipment

2 large bowls

Wooden spoon

Silicone spatula

Cutting board (optional)

Towel

Baking sheet

Parchment paper

Paring knife

Pastry brush

Small bowl

dough with your hands for 10 minutes. Press down with the heel of your hand, then fold the dough in half. Press down again and fold. Repeat.

3. **Let the dough rise.** When the dough changes from sticky to silky, place it in the greased bowl. Lay a clean towel over the bowl and set it in a warm spot. Allow the dough to rise for 45 minutes.

4. **Get ready to bake.** Preheat the oven to 375°F. Line a baking sheet with parchment paper.

5. **Decorate the breadsticks.** Dump the dough back onto your cutting board or counter. Ask an adult to help cut the dough into 12 pieces. Use your hands to roll out each piece of dough until it's long and thin like a snake. Place the dough on the parchment-lined baking sheet. Decorate with herbs and other add-ons until your design is complete! Brush with olive oil to keep the herbs from burning in the oven.

6. **Bake the breadsticks.** Carefully put the baking sheet in the oven and bake for 10 to 12 minutes, until the breadsticks look just golden on the edges. Ask an adult to help remove the sheet from the oven. Let cool briefly before eating.

 TOP TIP

▶ Your dough needs to rise enough to double in size! Take a peek after about 30 minutes, and if it's not rising yet, move your covered bowl to a warmer spot in the house.

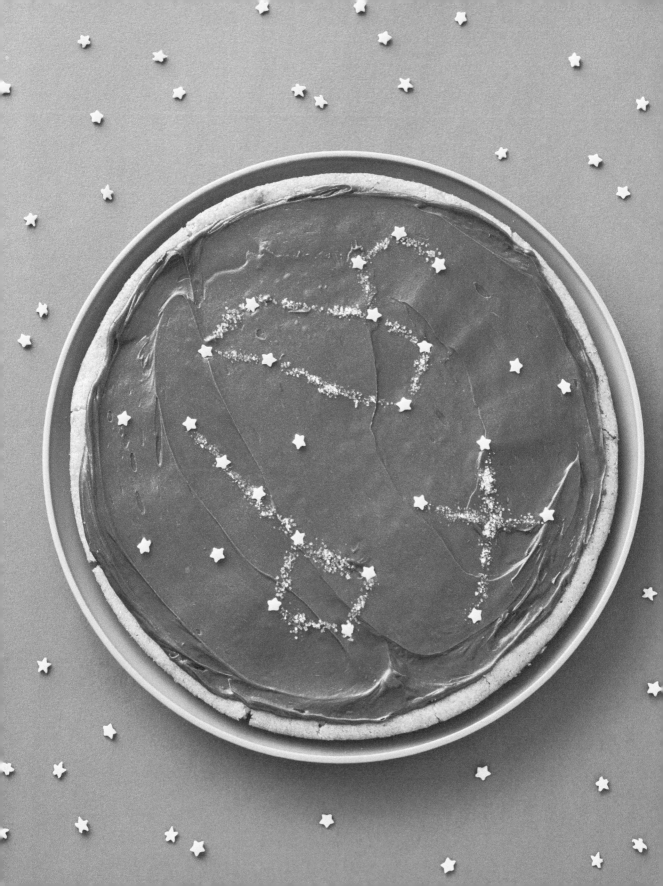

Constellation Cookie

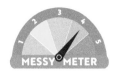

HARD

Nut-Free
Vegetarian

Prep time: 1 hour, plus
30 minutes to cool
Cook time: 20 minutes
Yield: 6 servings

Ingredients

Nonstick cooking spray

1 package refrigerated
sugar cookie dough

1 tub chocolate frosting

Gold star sprinkles

Golden sugar sprinkles

Tools/Equipment

Cast-iron skillet
or 9-inch round
baking pan

Kid-safe knife

You'll be seeing stars when you decorate this giant cookie with real constellations from the night sky! This design includes the Big Dipper, Leo, and the Southern Cross, but you can use the same idea to create any constellation you like.

1. **Get ready to bake.** Preheat the oven to 350°F. Coat a cast-iron skillet or 9-inch round baking pan with nonstick spray.

2. **Bake the cookie.** Spread out the cookie dough in a smooth, even layer inside the greased skillet. Carefully place the skillet in the oven and bake for 20 to 25 minutes, until the edges are golden. Ask an adult to help remove the skillet from the oven and set aside to cool completely, about 30 minutes.

3. **Frost the cookie.** Spread an even layer of chocolate frosting over the big cookie.

4. **Add the stars.** Use the gold stars to follow the design of these constellations or create one of your own! Finally, sprinkle the golden sugar sprinkles in between the stars to connect them.

TOP TIPS

▶ Be sure to let your cookie cool completely before you frost it!

▶ To make a flag with stars, you'll need a sticky note, a marker, a toothpick, and scissors. Fold the sticky note around the toothpick to seal it, then trim the edges with scissors. Use the marker to write the message.

▶ Instead of a big cookie, you could make 4 to 6 smaller cookies. They'll need to be big enough that you can design a constellation on top. Bake at 375°F for 10 to 12 minutes.

JUST FOR LAUGHS

What stars wear sunglasses? *Rock stars!*

How do astronauts hold up their pants? *With an asteroid belt!*

EXTRA CRAFTY

Do you know any other constellations? Ask a grown-up to help you look up a few others and draw out their shapes here!

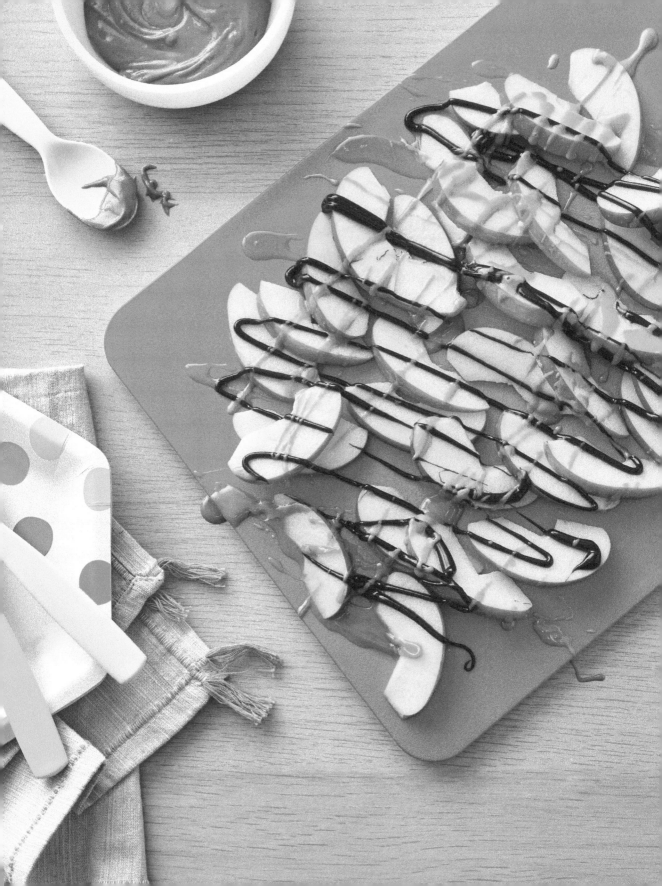

Pop Art Apple Nachos

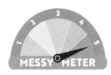

MEDIUM

Vegetarian

Prep time: 10 minutes
Cook time: 3 minutes
Yield: 4 servings

Ingredients

3 apples, sliced

⅓ cup nut butter

⅓ cup caramel sauce

⅓ cup fudge sauce

Tools/Equipment

Apple corer (optional)

Paring knife

3 small microwave-
safe bowls

Cutting board or plate

With zigs and zags, you'll design a gorgeous plate full of sweet and crunchy apple nachos in minutes! We like a combination of peanut butter, caramel, and fudge sauce, but you can use any kind of sauces you like. (If you want to get really fancy, add sprinkles!)

1. **Slice the apples.** Ask an adult to help core the apples and slice into wedges.

2. **Heat the sauces.** Put the nut butter, caramel sauce, and fudge sauce in 3 separate bowls. Ask an adult to help microwave each bowl individually until the ingredients are slightly liquefied, about 15 seconds each. (Use 3 small bowls if needed.)

3. **Get artsy!** Arrange the apple slices in a single layer on a cutting board or plate, keeping them as close together as possible. Drizzle the nut butter, caramel, and fudge sauce over the top.

→

TOP TIPS

▶ Homemade Caramel Sauce: Make your own 1-ingredient caramel sauce by placing an unopened can of sweetened condensed milk in a slow cooker and covering with water. Cover and cook on low for 3 hours. Open the can to find your milk has turned to caramel sauce!

▶ Homemade Fudge Sauce: Make your own fudge sauce by combining 1 cup sugar, 1 cup heavy cream, 1 cup unsweetened cocoa powder, and 4 tablespoons unsalted butter in a pot over medium heat. Stir until the butter melts and the sauce looks rich and creamy. This takes only a few minutes! Pour into jars and store in the refrigerator. When ready to use, heat in the microwave to liquefy.

DID YOU KNOW?

▶ Apples are a member of the rose family.

▶ Apples float because they're one-quarter air!

JUST FOR LAUGHS

How do you make an apple turnover?
Push it down a hill!

Who's an apple's favorite relative? *A granny!*

Why did the apple cry? *Because her peelings were hurt.*

EXTRA CRAFTY

Besides zigzags, what other kind of pattern could you make with the sauces? Draw your idea in the space below.

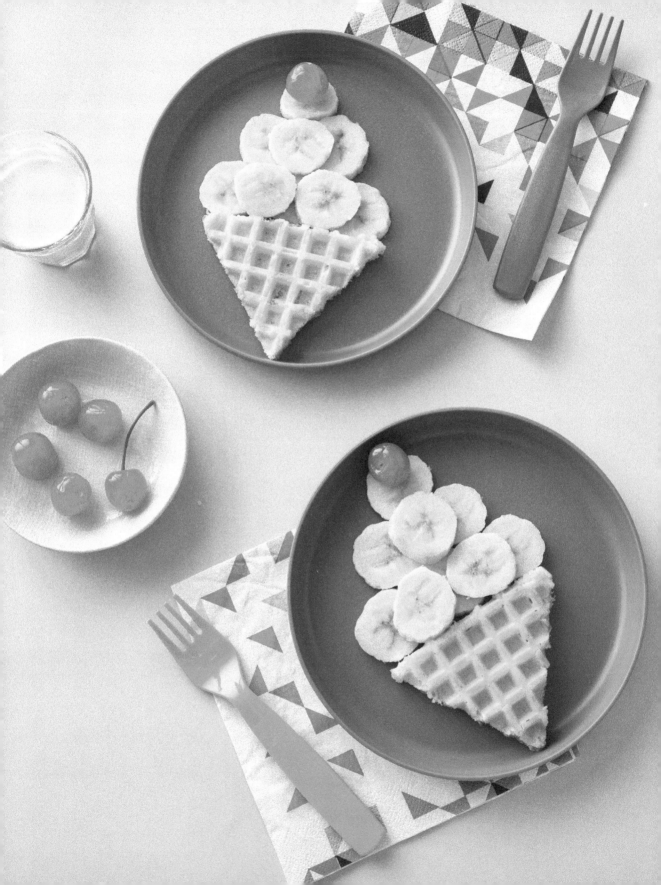

After-School Ice Cream Cones

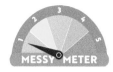

EASY

Dairy-Free Nut-Free
Vegetarian

Prep time: 5 minutes
Cook time: 3 minutes
Yield: 1 cone

Ingredients

1 frozen waffle

1 banana

1 maraschino cherry

Tools/Equipment

Toaster

Paring knife

Cutting board

Kid-safe knife

Plate

Put a new spin on plain ol' waffles with this banana-topped treat! Making more than one of these afternoon snacks? Double or triple the ingredients until you have enough for everyone.

1. **Toast the waffle.** Pop the waffle into the toaster and toast until it's defrosted and golden brown.

2. **Trim the waffle.** Ask an adult to help trim the edges off the waffle so that it becomes a triangle.

3. **Slice the bananas.** Peel the banana and use a kid-safe knife to slice it.

4. **Assemble the ice cream cone.** Place your waffle on a plate, then add 2 layers of banana slices in the shape of an ice cream scoop. Finish with a cherry on top.

TOP TIPS

▶ Want to make your own healthy-ish waffles? Use this super simple recipe from Foodlets.com: In a bowl, combine 1 cup whole wheat flour, 1 cup all-purpose flour, ¼ cup sugar, 2 tablespoons chia seeds, 4 teaspoons baking powder, ½ teaspoon salt, 2 large eggs, 2 cups vanilla yogurt, ½ cup vegetable or olive oil, ¼ cup water, and 1 teaspoon vanilla extract and mix well. Cook individual portions in a waffle iron until golden brown, about 4 minutes.

▶ Do you love bananas? Add a third or fourth layer of banana slices to make your "ice cream scoop" extra fluffy.

▶ Out of bananas? This idea works with sliced pineapple too.

DID YOU KNOW?

▶ The birth of the waffle dates to the Middle Ages, when they were cooked over a fire using two metal plates with wooden handles.

▶ The Waffle House restaurant chain sells 134 waffles a minute!

▶ Banana plants are not trees but rather a type of herb.

▶ Bananas can float in water.

JUST FOR LAUGHS

How do you make waffles smile? *Butter them up!*

How is baseball like waffles? *They both need good batters.*

EXTRA CRAFTY

What other shapes can you make out of waffles? Draw your idea in the space below!

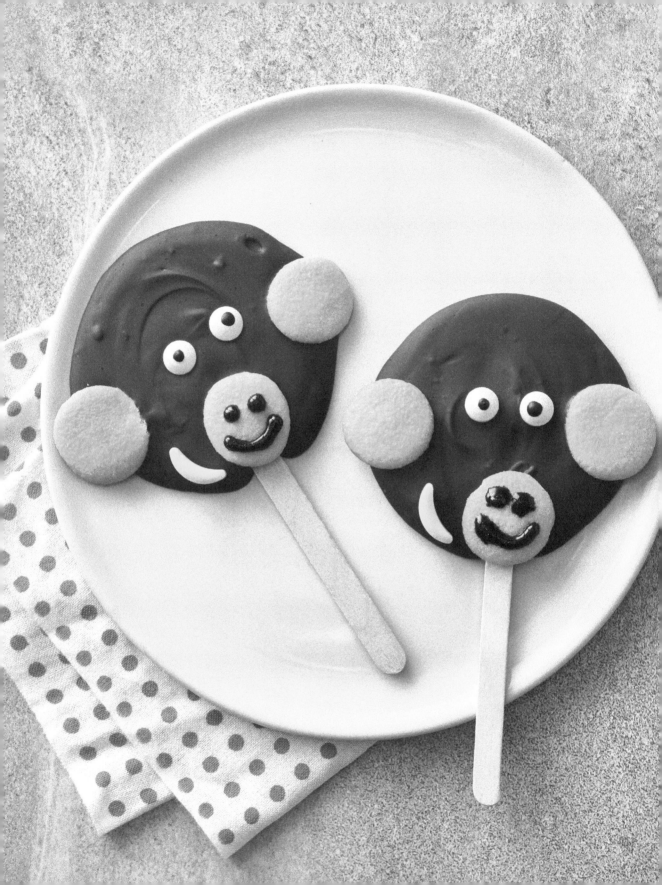

Curious George Chocolate Pops

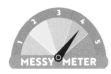

MEDIUM

Nut-Free   Vegetarian

Prep time: 15 minutes, plus 10 minutes to set
Yield: 1 pop

Ingredients

¼ cup chocolate chips or half a plain chocolate candy bar

3 mini vanilla cookies, such as Mini Nilla Wafers

1 tube black writing frosting

2 candy eyeballs

1 banana-shaped candy, such as Runts

Tools/Equipment

Microwave-safe bowl

Baking sheet

Parchment paper

Wooden craft sticks

Curious George never looked so cute! These homemade chocolate pops are simple to make and even more fun for a crowd to do together. The recipe below guides you through creating 1 pop. Making lots of pops? Double, triple, or even quadruple the ingredients until you have enough for everyone.

1. **Melt the chocolate.** Put the chocolate in a microwave-safe bowl. Ask an adult to help melt the chocolate in the microwave until it's pourable, in bursts of 10 seconds, stirring in between.

2. **Pour the chocolate.** Line a baking sheet with parchment paper. Carefully pour the chocolate onto the parchment paper in a round shape, about 4 inches wide. Insert the top of a wooden stick near the bottom of the circle, then flip it over so that both sides of the stick are coated with melted chocolate.

3. **Make a monkey face.** Draw a monkey nose and mouth on 1 vanilla cookie, using the black writing frosting. Add the eyes to your chocolate pop, then 2 plain ➜

vanilla cookies to the side of each eye for the ears. Place the cookie with the nose and mouth just below the eyes. Add the banana candy wherever you like!

4. **Allow to set.** Put the baking sheet in the refrigerator for about 10 minutes, until the chocolate is set (or let it firm up at room temperature for about 30 minutes).

TOP TIPS

▶ These pops are best to eat the day you make them. That way the cookies stay fresh.

▶ This technique works for lots of designs! Use pink candy melts instead of chocolate and top with sprinkles for a whole new look.

JUST FOR LAUGHS
What do you call an angry monkey?
Furious George.

EXTRA CRAFTY

You can create almost any design with this idea! What other colors, animals, or shapes could you make? Draw a picture of what you want to try next time in the space below.

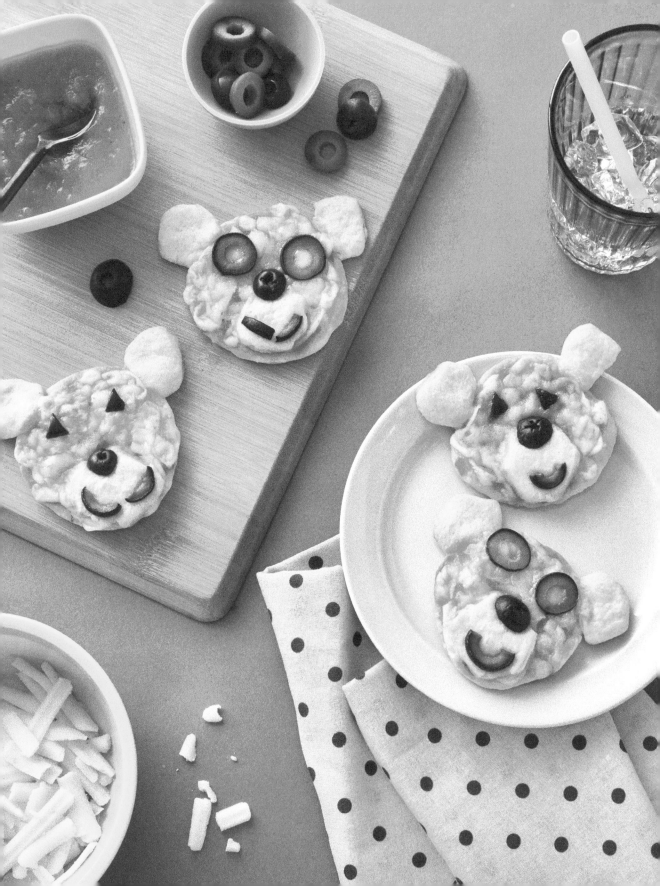

A Beary Good Day for Pizza

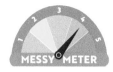

MEDIUM

Nut-Free Vegetarian

Prep time: 10 minutes
Cook time: 10 minutes
Yield: 4 small pizzas

Ingredients

1 small can sliced black olives, drained

1 tube crescent rolls

1 cup marinara sauce

2 cups shredded mozzarella cheese

Tools/Equipment

Baking sheet

Parchment paper

Paring knife

Cutting board

Spoon

How do you make everyone's favorite food even better? Add the cutest face you've ever seen on a baking sheet! These little bears come together quickly and cook faster than a full-size pizza. You'll have plenty of pizza to snack on in minutes. Bonus: They store well in the refrigerator, so you can save some for tomorrow's lunch box.

1. **Get ready to bake.** Preheat the oven to 350°F. Line a baking sheet with parchment paper.

2. **Use olives for the face.** Ask an adult to help cut some sliced olives in half, or into small pieces, for the eyes and nose.

3. **Cut circles in the dough.** Open the can of dough. Ask an adult to help cut round pieces, as large as you can make them. Save the scraps of dough.

4. **Make the ears.** Put the dough circles on the parchment-lined baking sheet. For each bear, roll 2 small pieces of the dough scraps into balls to make the ears. Place the balls near the top of each big circle. Press down gently, making sure you flatten the dough and connect the pieces together.

→

5. **Add the toppings.** Use a spoon to gently add marinara sauce to each bear face. Top with a sprinkle of mozzarella cheese. Then add the olives for the eyes and a nose.

6. **Bake.** Ask an adult to carefully put the baking sheet in the oven and bake for 6 to 8 minutes, until the dough looks golden on the edges and the cheese has melted. Ask an adult to help remove the baking sheet from the oven. Let the pizzas cool for a bit before eating.

TOP TIPS

▶ Use a large round cookie cutter if you have one. If not, tracing around the edges of the olive can works too!

▶ The olives will probably move a bit during the baking process when the cheese melts. You may need to scooch them back into place when the pizzas come out of the oven.

JUST FOR LAUGHS

What did the teddy bear say after dinner?
I'm stuffed.

What do you call a wet bear? *A drizzly bear!*

DID YOU KNOW?

▶ Teddy bears are named after President Theodore Roosevelt, who loved the outdoors. He refused to shoot a bear that his friends had captured during a hunting trip in 1902, and the story made him a hero.

▶ Bears are big and heavy, but they can still run very fast! They're also good at climbing and swimming.

▶ Winnie-the-Pooh was a real bear, and a female! As a cub, she was adopted by a Canadian soldier, who named her Winnipeg after his hometown. She traveled with the Canadian army during World War I until eventually he brought her to the London Zoo. That's where a little boy named Christopher Robin fell in love with her. His father, a writer named A. A. Milne, was so inspired that he created the entire Winnie-the-Pooh series.

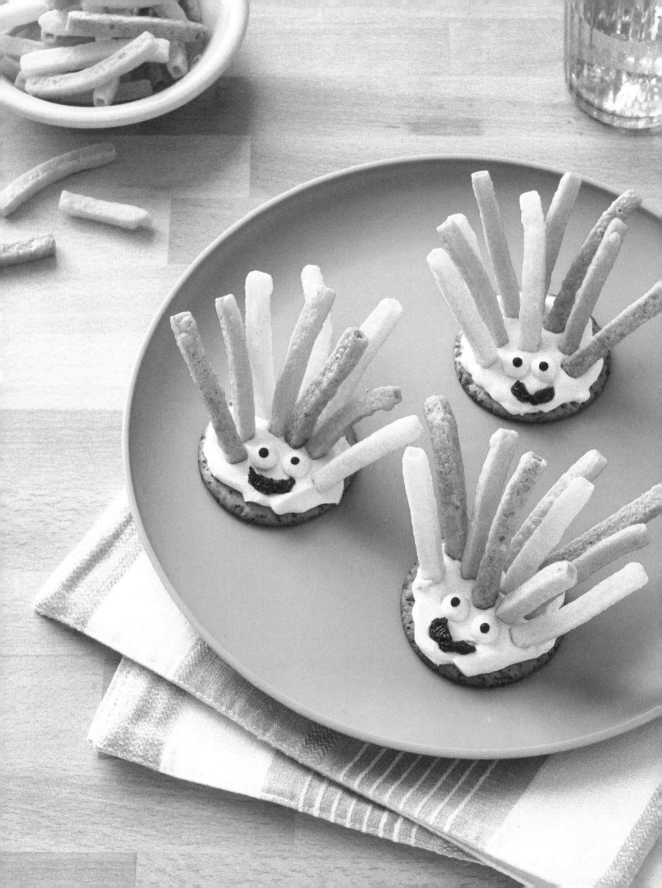

Crazy Hair, Just Don't Care

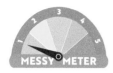

EASY

Nut-Free Vegetarian

Prep time: 5 minutes
Yield: 1 serving

Ingredients

1 tablespoon
cream cheese

1 large round cracker
(about 3 inches)

1 raisin

2 candy eyes

12 veggie straws

Tools/Equipment

Kid-safe knife

Paring knife

Cutting board

Who knew wild hair could be so tasty? Crunch your way through snack time with these kooky crackers. Use any kind of cream cheese or nut butter you like for the "glue." Veggie straws work great for hair, but I bet you can think of other fun ideas too! You can even draw a picture right here in this book. In the meantime, double or triple the ingredients listed below to create more than one crazy hair snack.

1. **Set the "glue."** Use a kid-safe knife to gently spread the cream cheese on the cracker. It should be thick enough to hold the veggie straws in place.

2. **Make a face.** Ask an adult to help cut a raisin in half lengthwise to make a mouth. Roll one raisin half in your palms to shape it into half a circle. (You can eat the other half!) (Half a raisin is easier to shape, plus you can eat the other piece!) Place the candy eyes and the raisin mouth at the bottom of your cream cheese–covered cracker.

→

3. **Add the hair.** Poke the veggie straws into the cream cheese to cover the rest of the cracker. Mix and match colors and directions or make a pattern. It's up to you!

DID YOU KNOW?

▶ Cream cheese is a soft, white cheese made either with cream or with a mixture of milk and cream. It's different from other cheeses because it's not aged at all.

▶ Speaking of age, cream cheese isn't new. It was enjoyed in England as far back as 1583!

▶ Crackers are typically made in factories. The dough starts out as extra-large sheets in thin layers. Pins press holes into the sheets of dough, then they are baked in big ovens.

▶ Veggie straws are closer to potato chips than you might think! They're usually a puffed-up mixture of potato flour, sunflower oil, and cornstarch. Then flavors are added, often including tomato puree, spinach powder, salt, sugar, and turmeric.

JUST FOR LAUGHS

Where do sheep get their hair cut? *At the baa-baa shop!*

One friend said, "I'm getting my hair cut today." The other friend warned, "You should get them all cut. Otherwise it'll look funny!"

EXTRA CRAFTY

What other fun hair can you give your snack? Draw it here!

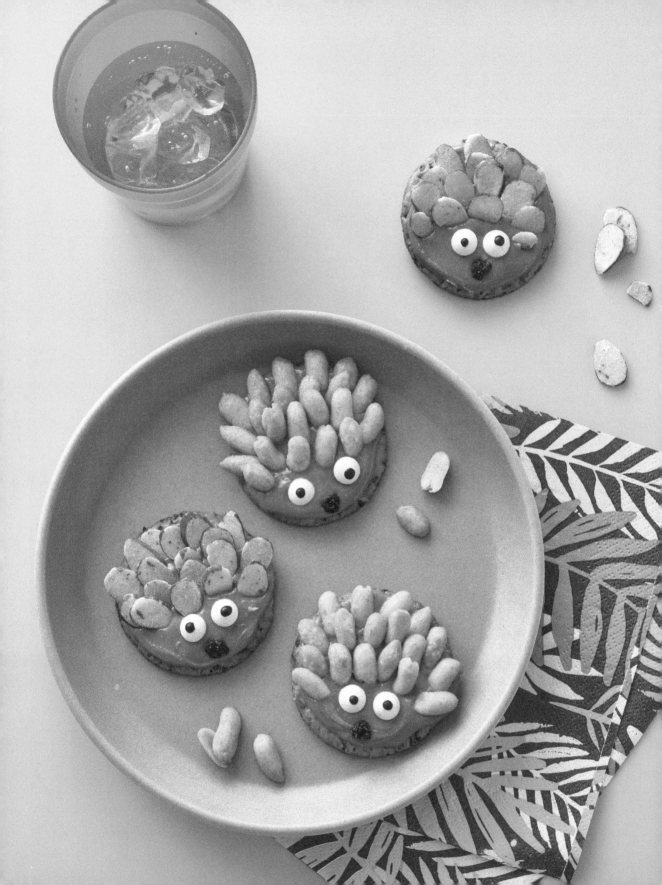

Peanut the Hedgehog Cracker

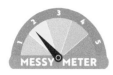

MEDIUM

Dairy-Free
Vegetarian

Prep time: 5 minutes
Yield: 1 serving

Ingredients

1 tablespoon peanut
butter or almond butter

1 large round cracker
(about 3 inches)

1 raisin

2 candy eyes

25 to 30 peanut halves
or almond slivers

Tools/Equipment

Kid-safe knife

Paring knife

Cutting board

*What's brown and pointy and delicious all over?
This adorable hedgehog snack! Grab a cracker
and a handful of peanuts to get started. The
materials here are everything you need to make
one hedgehog. Double or triple (or keep going) to
have enough to make with a group of friends.*

1. **Set the "glue."** Use a kid-safe knife to
   gently spread the peanut butter on the
   cracker. It should be thick enough to
   hold the peanuts in place.

2. **Make a face.** Ask an adult to help cut
   a raisin in half lengthwise to make a
   mouth. Roll one raisin half in your palms
   to shape it into a circle. (You can eat the
   other half!) Place the candy eyes and
   raisin mouth at the bottom of the peanut
   butter–covered cracker.

3. **Add the spikes.** Poke the peanuts into
   the peanut butter to cover the rest of
   the cracker.

TOP TIPS

- ▶ No candy eyes? Use M&Ms or more raisins.
- ▶ If peanuts are a no-go, use almonds and almond butter instead.

DID YOU KNOW?

- ▶ January 24 is National Peanut Butter Day.
- ▶ According to one survey, the average American will eat almost 3,000 peanut butter sandwiches in their lifetime!
- ▶ Two peanut farmers have been elected president of the United States: Thomas Jefferson from Virginia and Jimmy Carter from Georgia.
- ▶ A group of hedgehogs is called an array.
- ▶ Hedgehogs rely on their noses and ears because they have very poor eyesight.
- ▶ Hedgehogs have between 5,000 and 7,000 quills!

JUST FOR LAUGHS

Where do hedgehog wizards learn spells?

At Hedgehog-warts.

EXTRA CRAFTY

What friends does Peanut the Hedgehog have? Draw what they look like here!

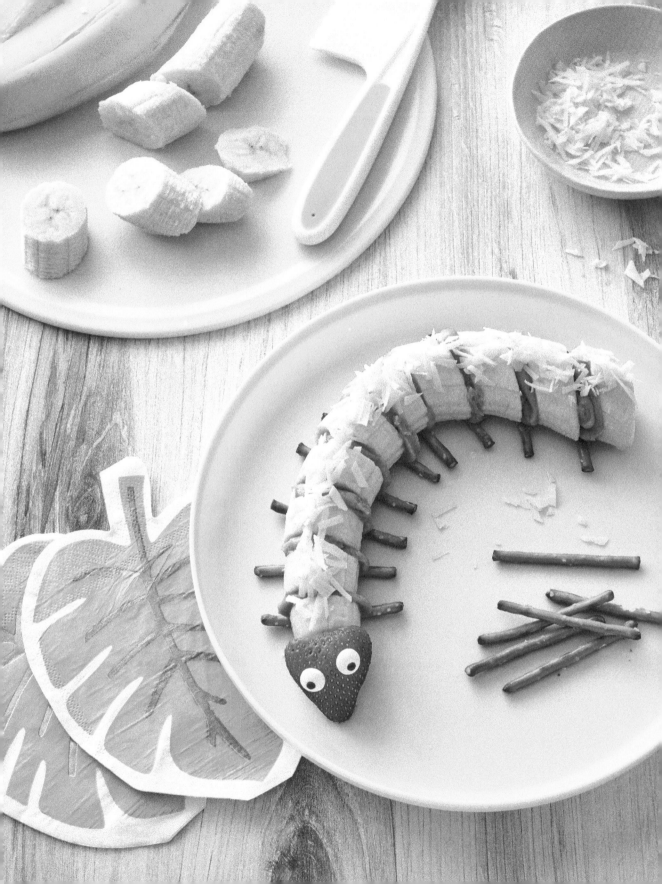

Fuzzy Wuzzy Caterpillar

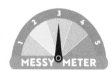

MEDIUM

Dairy-Free
Vegetarian

Prep time: 10 minutes
Yield: 1 serving

Ingredients

1 banana

12 pretzel sticks

¼ cup peanut butter or nut butter

1 strawberry

2 candy eyes

1 tablespoon sweet-ened coconut flakes

Tools/Equipment

Kid-safe knife

Cutting board

Plate

Paring knife

Inching along, right onto your plate! This sweet and satisfying caterpillar is almost as fun to make as it is delicious to eat. The ingredients here make a single caterpillar. Luckily with this recipe it's easy to make as many snacks as you need!

1. **Slice the banana.** Peel the banana. Use a kid-safe knife to cut off the ends of the banana (snack!), then cut the banana into slices about 1 inch wide.

2. **Arrange the legs.** Place pretzel sticks on the plate in the shape you want your caterpillar to be. (Don't worry, you can move them later if you need to.)

3. **Set the "glue."** Use the kid-safe knife to spread peanut butter between the banana slices, then stick the whole thing together and arrange it on the plate, right on top of the pretzel stick legs. Make your caterpillar a C shape or more of an S. It's up to you!

4. **Make a face.** Ask an adult to help cut off the stem and hull from the strawberry. Use peanut butter to glue the strawberry in front of the banana. Glue the eyes on the front of your strawberry.

5. **Add the fuzz.** Sprinkle coconut flakes over the top.

TOP TIPS

▶ Give this caterpillar a new look (and taste) by substituting sprinkles for the coconut and cream cheese for the peanut butter!

▶ Get more advanced by gluing sliced raisins above the eyes for eyebrows!

DID YOU KNOW?

▶ Bananas ripen best when they're picked green.

▶ The way caterpillars move is unique. No other animals move like they do, in a wave motion, starting in back and moving up to the front.

▶ Caterpillars have 12 eyes.

▶ It looks like caterpillars have tons of legs, but since they are insects, they only have 6 real legs. The rest are called "false legs." They are arms with tiny hooks on the ends to help with walking and climbing.

EXTRA CRAFTY

Take a moment to think about what you've made! What is your favorite craft so far? Draw what you've created here!

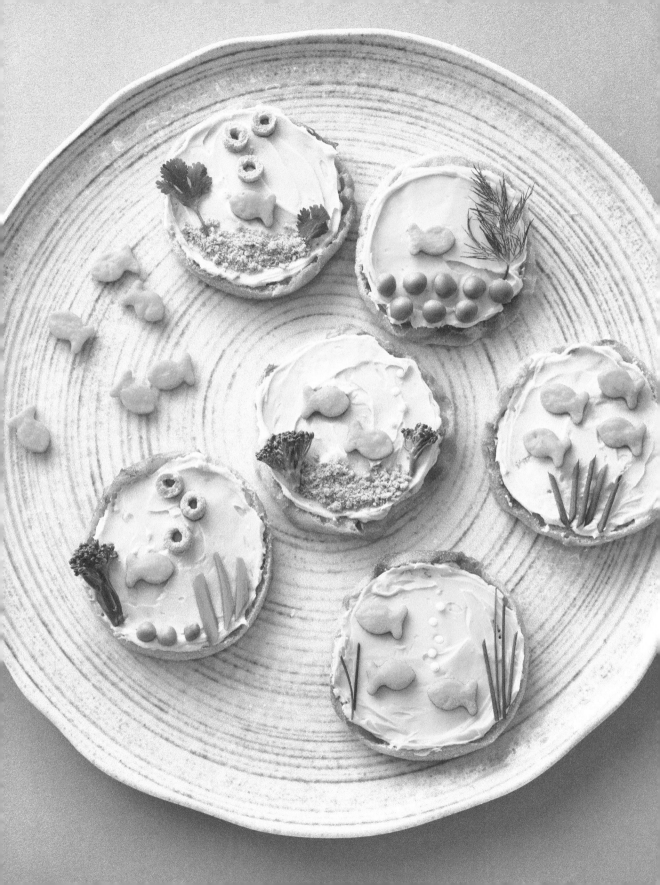

Under the Sea Snacks

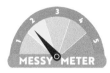

EASY

Nut-Free

Vegetarian

Prep time: 10 minutes
Yield: 12 snacks

Ingredients

6 English muffins

Blue food coloring

6 ounces cream cheese, at room temperature

Fish-shaped crackers, such as Goldfish

Fresh herbs and cut-up veggies, such as carrot sticks and small broccoli florets

Crushed graham crackers (optional)

Large white sprinkles or O-shaped cereal, such as Cheerios (optional)

Tools/Equipment

Toaster

Food processor or bowl and silicone spatula

Kid-safe knife

Fire up the toaster and raid the cupboards for a crunchy, sweet snack that will fill you up with one of the most popular crackers around! Use whatever veggies or herbs you have. Your imagination is the key ingredient. This is a fun snack to make with friends, since you'll have plenty of ingredients to feed a crowd. Plan enough time to create—and enjoy—your snacks since these are best to eat right away.

When you're all finished, share your creation! Take a photo and use hashtag #LittleFoodies on social media.

1. **Toast the English muffins.** Split the English muffins, then toast them until golden brown.

2. **Create the sea.** Ask an adult to help use a small food processor to blend 2 or 3 drops of blue food coloring into the cream cheese (or do it yourself with a bowl and spatula). Mix until you like the color.

3. **Add "water."** Use a kid-safe knife to spread blue cream cheese all over each English muffin half.

→

4. **Assemble the fish's home.** Place fish crackers in the middle and arrange the herbs and veggies around them to create sea plants. If you're using crushed graham crackers, put those at the bottom, like sand. If you have white sprinkles or cereal O's, add them above the fish, like air bubbles.

TOP TIPS

▶ No English muffins? Use graham crackers as your ocean background.

▶ Celebrating Shark Week? Swap the fish crackers for gummy sharks!

DID YOU KNOW?

▶ English muffins aren't really popular in England! Just like French fries don't really come from France, this is another name Americans use. If you go to England and want something similar to an English muffin, it's better to ask for a "crumpet."

▶ The part of broccoli you eat is actually baby flowers that haven't opened yet. Once the flowers open, the broccoli tastes bitter.

▶ Goldfish crackers started out as a snack in Switzerland before becoming a popular treat all over the world.

▶ Even astronauts like Goldfish crackers! The space shuttle *Discovery* packed these snacks on their mission in 1988.

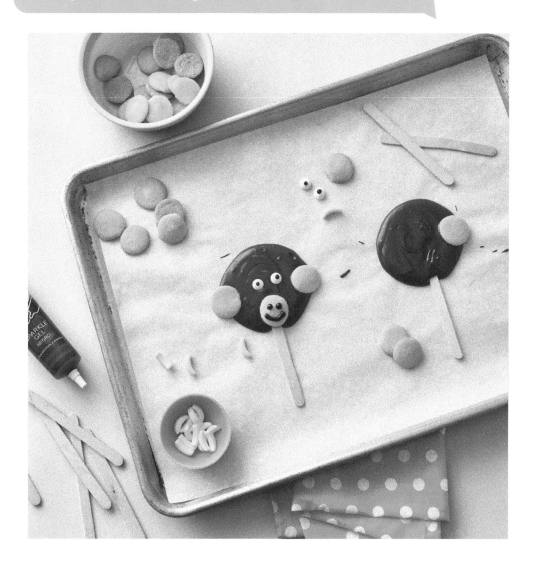

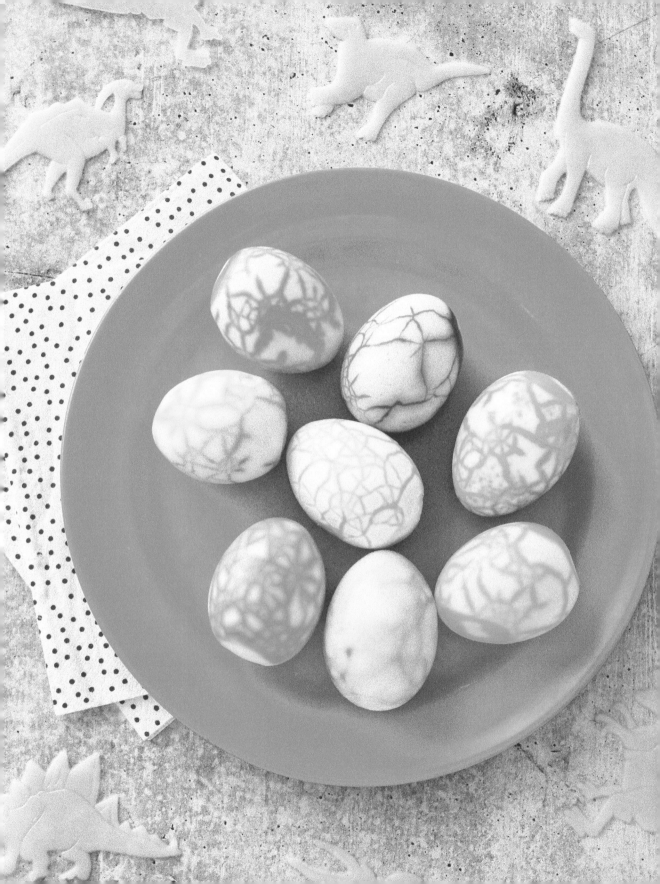

Prehistoric Dino Eggs

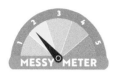

HARD

Nut-Free
Gluten-Free
Vegetarian

Prep time: 15 minutes, plus 4 hours to set
Cook time: 15 minutes
Yield: 6 eggs

Ingredients

6 eggs

Food coloring in 6 colors

Tools/Equipment

Large saucepan

Large bowl

6 mugs

Take your hard-boiled egg game to the next level—and another time period—with these colorful eggs that look like they came right out of the prehistoric age! Just keep in mind that these need to set, so you'll need to make your eggs the day before you want to eat them. Use any kind of eggs you like: white or brown. The color of the shell doesn't matter. Just wait until you see the color inside. That's where the real fun begins!

1. **Boil the eggs.** Ask an adult to help boil the eggs. This is my favorite method for making hard-boiled eggs: Put the eggs in a saucepan and cover them with about an inch of water. Bring to a boil. Turn off the burner. Cover the pan and allow the eggs to sit for 12 minutes. Carefully transfer the eggs to a bowl of ice-cold water to stop the cooking. Don't peel them! (Note: You can do this step up to 3 days ahead of time and refrigerate the hard-boiled eggs until you're ready for step 2.)

2. **Prepare to color.** Fill each mug halfway with water and add a few drops of food coloring to each one, using a different color for each mug.

3. **Crack the eggs.** Gently tap the boiled eggs on the counter in a few places until they start to crack, but don't peel them! Roll them in your hand a little, just to make sure you have lots of cracks all over.

4. **Dye the eggs.** Place 1 egg in each coloring mug until it's submerged. (Not enough liquid? Add more water and another drop or two of color.) Carefully put the mugs in the refrigerator and let the eggs sit for at least 4 hours or as long as 12 hours; the longer they sit, the more color you'll get.

5. **Peel.** Remove the eggs from the mugs and rinse with water so that you don't get coloring all over your hands. Reveal each egg's cool pattern by gently peeling the eggs!

 ## DID YOU KNOW?

▶ Not sure if that egg in your refrigerator is hard-boiled or raw? Try spinning it. Hard-boiled eggs spin smoothly. If it's wobbling, that's because the liquid inside is shifting around and it's most likely raw.

▶ Paleontologists believe that, depending on the species, female dinosaurs laid up to 15 or 20 eggs in a single sitting!

▶ Chickens of different breeds can lay eggs with different colored shells, including brown, blue, and even green. But all eggs look the same inside.

▶ Think you found a dinosaur egg at your house? Experts say this is very, very rare. Unless other dinosaur bones have been found nearby, it's probably a fossilized chicken egg but could still be around 100 years old.

JUST FOR LAUGHS

What do you call a dinosaur wearing a cowboy hat? *Tyrannosaurus Tex!*

What do you call a dinosaur's ghost? *A scary-dactyl!*

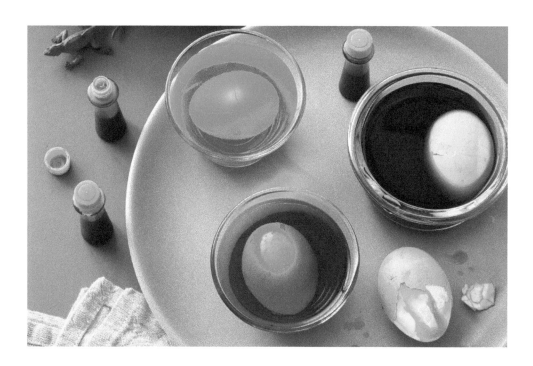

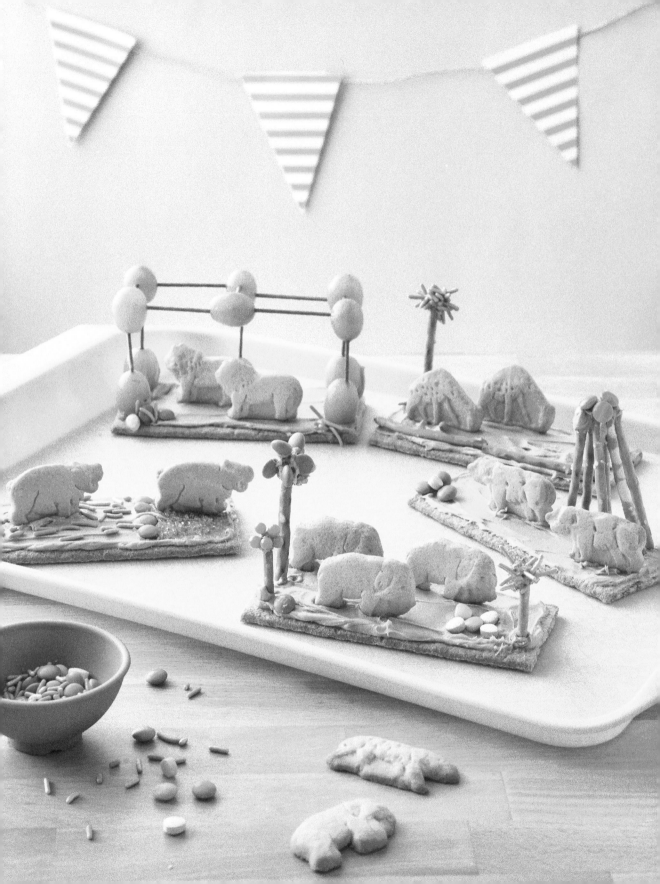

Animal Crackers at the Zoo

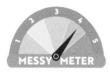

HARD

Vegetarian

Prep time: 45 minutes
Yield: 6 to 8 servings

Ingredients

6 ounces cream cheese, at room temperature

2 tablespoons maple syrup

Green food coloring

Blue food coloring

2 to 3 tablespoons peanut butter

2 sleeves graham crackers

4 (2.13 ounce) boxes animal crackers

Veggie straws or pretzel sticks

Add-ons, such as gold and blue sprinkles, colored sprinkles, assorted gummy candies, and fruit-shaped candies like Runts

8 ounces grapes

The perfect snack to make with friends, this zoo scene comes to life with sweetened cream cheese and all the zoo accessories you can think of! It's the most complicated—and maybe the most fun—project in the whole book. Start with animal crackers and stop when your imagination runs out.

1. **Color the "glue."** In a large bowl, combine the cream cheese and maple syrup. Transfer one-quarter of the mixture to a small bowl. To the small bowl, add 2 to 3 drops of blue food coloring and mix it in. This is the water for your animals' habitats. To the large bowl, add 2 to 6 drops of green food coloring and mix it in. This is the grass for your zoo. The peanut butter will be sand or dirt. Spread a thick layer of green, blue, or brown "glue" on each graham cracker and place them on a baking sheet.

2. **Arrange the animals.** Sort through each package of animal crackers and make sets of matching animals: all the giraffes in one pile, all the elephants, and so on. Arrange the animals so that they're →

Tools/Equipment

Large bowl

Silicone spatula

Small bowl

Baking sheet or large serving tray

Toothpicks

Sticky notes (optional)

Scissors (optional)

Marker (optional)

standing upright in their appropriate habitats (grass, water, or sand).

3. **Set up the habitats.** Use the veggie straws or pretzel sticks to make trees, and the other candies to make borders for each species's home.

4. **Make the monkey cage.** Start by putting down a layer of either cream cheese or peanut butter. Now it's time to build a cage of toothpicks secured by grapes. If you need to, refer to the Write Your Name in Grapes project (page 41) for help with this technique. Once that's done, place the monkeys in their cages!

5. **Make signs (optional).** Use the technique from our Constellation Cookie project (page 65) to make signs for each exhibit: Fold a sticky note around a toothpick to seal it, then trim the edges with scissors. Write the name of the habitat on the flag. Poke it into the cream cheese or peanut butter.

DID YOU KNOW?

▶ Animal crackers were made in England as early as the 17th century.

▶ Barnum's Animals is the most popular brand of animal crackers in America. Each box contains 22 crackers featuring up to 19 different animals.

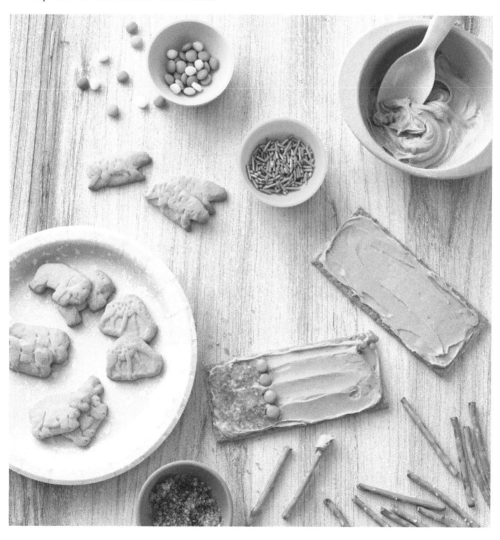

INDEX

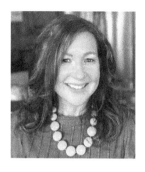

Charity Mathews is a former executive at Martha Stewart and HGTV who's now a family food writer at foodlets.com. That's where you'll find her super simple recipes packed with fresh ingredients and tried-and-true advice about raising little foodies. She's been featured on foodnetwork.com, Huffington Post, WHUP radio, ABC 11-TV, and more. The author of four additional cookbooks for kids, Charity lives on a small farm in North Carolina with her family of six, plus their rescue dogs, bunnies, chickens, and bees.

CPSIA information can be obtained
at www.ICGtesting.com
Printed in the USA
LVHW071744170322
713720LV00007B/228